T0364691

Sociological Approaches to Health, Healthcare and Nursing

Sociological Approaches to Health, Healthcare and Nursing

A Critical Introduction

HANNAH COOKE, BSc, MSc (Econ), MSc (Nurs), PhD, RGN, NDN, RNT

Honorary Senior Lecturer
Division of Nursing
Midwifery and Social Work
School of Health Sciences
University of Manchester
Manchester, United Kingdom

ELSEVIER

SOCIOLOGICAL APPROACHES TO HEALTH, HEALTHCARE AND NURSING: A CRITICAL INTRODUCTION

Notice

ISBN: 978-0-702-08314-3

Executive Content Strategist: Robert Edwards
Content Project Manager: Shruti Raj
Design: Standard
Illustration Manager: Christian Bilbow
Marketing Manager: Belinda Tudin

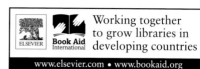

Working together to grow libraries in developing countries

Printed in India
Last digit is the print number: 9 8 7 6 5 4 3 2 1

www.elsevier.com • www.bookaid.org

PREFACE

This book provides a critical introduction to sociology of health and illness. It is aimed, particularly, at nurses and other health and social care professionals. It has a particular focus on inequalities of health and the institutional practices that sustain them. I have described it as a 'critical' introduction because it invites readers to look critically at their own practice and at the institutional context in which they work. For example, it critically examines some fashionable healthcare concepts such as patient self-care. The book introduces readers to some key sociological theories and concepts and encourages readers to think of these as tools which can help them to examine the institutional, social and cultural environment in which they practice.

The first UK nursing regulator (the General Nursing Council (GNC)) first recommended that social sciences should be taught to nurses in 1923. That recommendation was repeated by the GNC soon after the creation of the NHS in 1953, and successive regulators have reiterated it since. It was suggested in 1953 that sociology could help nurses to see the patient as a 'whole person'. It has now been more than a hundred years since the need for nurses to have some understanding of sociology was first recognised. However, there is still considerable variation in the teaching of sociology to nurses and other health professionals and still some ambivalence towards sociological knowledge amongst some members of the nursing and medical professions. In Chapter 1, I explain the value of the sociology of health and illness to health professionals. I hope that this book will show the reader how this branch of sociology can help us to understand the context of our practice.

When I left school, I studied for a degree in sociology at the London School of Economics. I had to suspend my studies in my third year to care for my terminally ill mother. After her death, I took a job as a nursing assistant on the old age psychiatry ward of a local hospital while studying to finish my degree on my days off. It was these experiences that led me to understand the value of nursing. It was, above all, nurses who made a difference when I was caring for my mother at home at the end of her life. As a result, I decided to choose nursing as a career. I first studied the sociology of health and illness shortly after this by undertaking a master's degree in 'sociology as applied to medicine' at Bedford College, University of London. I completed this course while waiting for a nurse training place at the Royal London Hospital. I met some inspiring teachers of sociology of health and illness at this time; not least, Margot Jefferys. Margot was a woman of great compassion who had pioneered teaching and research on what was then called 'medical sociology' in the UK. Sir Michael Marmot, whose groundbreaking work has shaped our understanding of health inequalities, was an inspirational visiting lecturer. You will meet his work in this book.

During my clinical nursing career, I worked in acute medicine, intensive care, palliative care and primary care, both within a GP practice and as a district nurse. To me, it was always clear that people's social circumstances were central to their experience of illness and their chance of getting better. This was particularly evident when working in primary care where I was often caring for people living incredibly difficult lives due to factors beyond their control. Thus, my clinical experiences continually demonstrated to me the relevance of sociology of health and illness to understanding patients' lives and healthcare experiences.

My clinical experience also came in a variety of different institutional contexts, each with its own structure and culture. I learnt that some workplaces were supportive and helped staff to deliver high-quality care while other settings had different priorities, such as saving money or speeding up episodes of care. I quickly realised that good care needs good support. I have since carried out research into failures in care, and these issues are addressed in the later chapters of the book. Thus, this book takes a critical look at health policy and politics and at healthcare institutions. It encourages readers to develop their own ideas about how our health services are organised and how they could be improved.

I have now spent many years in nurse education. I started by teaching students practical skills in clinical practice but then moved on to teaching and researching nursing at the University of Manchester. This included undertaking a PhD in sociology, examining nursing discipline and regulation, under the supervision of Professor Huw Beynon. Among my other teaching duties, I have taught sociology of health and illness to many generations of undergraduate and post-registration students in nursing and other health professions. This book brings together what I have learnt during my years of teaching sociology of health to health professionals.

I started planning this book with my good friend and colleague Dr Shaun Speed. Shaun had studied sociology at university some years after starting his career in nursing. For Shaun, too, the experience of working in the community had demonstrated the value of a sociological understanding of illness. Shaun and I had worked together teaching sociology to undergraduates both in the UK and in Singapore. We wrote the book proposal together, so Shaun played an important part in planning the structure and detailed content of the book. Unfortunately, ill health meant that Shaun was unable to work on the book we had planned, and so I undertook to carry on with the book alone. Sadly, Shaun died unexpectedly early in 2023. Shaun was a warm, funny and incredibly kind man who was deeply committed to his profession, his patients and his students. He was also passionately committed to social justice. I hope that this completed book does justice to his vision and to the book we initially planned together. This book is dedicated to his memory.

ACKNOWLEDGEMENTS

This book would never have happened without the initial involvement of my friend and work colleague, the late Dr Shaun Speed (see preface). Shaun played an important part in initiating this book, planning its content and writing the book proposal. His presence is much missed.

My thanks go to Professor Valerie Bryson for agreeing to review the chapter on gender and for her helpful and perceptive comments.

I am grateful to the initial commissioning editor of this book, Alison Taylor, for seeing the need for this book. I am also grateful to my editors, Robert Edwards and Shruti Raj, for their patience and support.

Finally, my thanks go to all my former students who have inspired me to complete this book.

DEDICATION

This book is dedicated to the memory of Dr Shaun Speed (1964–2023).

Inequalities and Social Determinants of Health

CHAPTER 1

Sociology of Health and Illness and the Social Determinants of Health

This chapter introduces the sociology of health and illness and outlines the reasons why a distinctively sociological approach to health and illness can be useful for health professionals. It briefly considers what is distinctive about sociology as a discipline and looks at how sociologists work. It then looks in more detail at models of illness and considers the importance of a sociological understanding of health and illness, particularly in the field of public health. It introduces the social determinants of health and considers how sociology helps us to 'think upstream' about the causes of ill health. The three sections of the book are briefly outlined.

Why Study Sociology of Health and Illness?

Some of the readers of this book will already be health professionals, while others of you will be just starting a career in healthcare. You may have a very clear idea of why you entered your profession and what your ambitions are for your future career, or you may still be finding your feet. In either case, you will be aware that your chosen field of work is rarely out of the media. You will have seen that there are many people out there with fierce ideas about what is wrong and right with healthcare systems such as the UK's National Health Service (NHS) and what the solutions should be. You may have also noticed that media debates about healthcare are often polarised. Some media voices hark back to an idealised past when there were still matrons in charge and nurses wore frilly hats and were expected to open doors for doctors. Other media pundits look forward to a bright technological future where digital technology will dominate healthcare, telemedicine will replace face-to-face contact with patients and bedside nurses will be replaced by robots.

The COVID-19 pandemic led to even more conflict and debate about healthcare than usual with fierce debates, in particular about the role of public health in our everyday lives, most notably amongst those politically opposed to vaccination. Some sociologists have suggested that we are living in an 'antiscience' and 'posttruth' era (Prasad, 2022). This highlights the new role of social media in providing health information or misinformation and in shaping health beliefs. You have entered a field of work that has become highly politicised in the last few decades. Unfortunately, many of the political debates about healthcare are noteworthy for being devoid of sound evidence.

You are also entering a rapidly changing field. Healthcare in the UK has been subject to a great deal of institutional turbulence with NHS organisations reorganised so frequently in the last four decades that the process has been described as a 'continuous revolution' (Webster, 2002). The roles of healthcare professionals have also changed radically in recent years, with new occupations being developed such as advanced practitioner, nurse associate and physician associate. At the same time, the boundaries between existing occupations such as doctors, nurses and healthcare assistants are being redrawn. You may be wondering just how different your chosen profession will be in the future or whether it will even exist at all. Some authors have even pessimistically forecast the 'demise' of nursing as a profession (Shields & Watson, 2007).

The lives of your patients have changed too. To give a few examples, we are currently experiencing a 'cost-of-living crisis' with deepening inequality and spiralling levels of poverty and destitution. This negatively impacts people's health as well as diminishing their resources to cope with illness. We also have a population who are living longer with more people working further into old age and facing new challenges to manage long-term illnesses alongside other demands. The number of people living alone has steadily increased, so there are more people facing illness with limited social support. There are new uncertainties about gender identity with more people dealing with the specific health challenges associated with being transgender or non-binary. Wars, climate change and famine around the world are having health-damaging effects and displacing large numbers of people, creating political conflicts about how to manage the increase in refugee populations. We face present and future challenges from climate change that both the government and the NHS have barely come to grips with (Harmer et al., 2020; Solomon & LaRocque, 2019). All of these social and cultural changes in society have an everyday impact on the work of health professionals, creating new demands and new challenges.

This book argues that health professionals need to have a critical understanding of the social, cultural and political landscape within which they work. The puzzles and challenges that we face in our working lives can be stressful if we do not have the tools to make sense of them. The book suggests that sociological ideas and evidence can help us to form this critical understanding. Sometimes it is important to stand back from the everyday pressures of our working lives and take stock of the situation we find ourselves in. For example, if we feel that we cannot deliver the high standards of care we aspire to due to a heavy workload, we may need to understand that this is not a problem of our own making. We are not 'failures' if we struggle to 'cope'. Instead we are experiencing institutional pressures which are the result of wider social and political forces, and in this we are not alone. Similarly, if we see our patients facing stigma or discrimination, or being given suboptimal care, we need to be able to look critically at why this has happened and at the social and institutional context which allowed this inadequate care to occur.

In the next section, we will look at the idea of the 'sociological imagination' and consider how this might enable us to develop a critical understanding of the world we live and work in.

The Sociological Imagination

The idea of the **'sociological imagination'** was first proposed by a mid–20th-century sociologist C. Wright Mills (Mills, 2000). Mills was a 'social conflict theorist' concerned about inequalities in society. Mills said that many of us experience 'private troubles' in our everyday lives such as losing a job, struggling to find a place to live, having difficulty finding the money to pay our bills, and feeling lonely or anxious. If we are nurses, we may experience work troubles such as feeling stressed and overworked or struggling to juggle family life and work. Too often, we blame ourselves and feel that we should be able to solve these problems ourselves by working harder, managing our time or finances better, taking better care of our mental health or having more 'resilience' (Traynor, 2018). This is certainly the message we are often fed by the media and by 'official' sources. Thus

Traynor has critiqued the management discourse that asks overworked nurses to learn 'resilience'. Mills takes a broader view of our private troubles seeing them as 'public issues' which reflect structural changes and inequalities in society. Mills says that the sociological imagination enables us to grasp 'history and biography' and see the relation between the two in society. It is only by recognising the structural roots of our 'private troubles' that we can confront the social, political and economic conditions that have caused them.

Giddens (1986) says that the sociological imagination is achieved by exercising the imagination in three ways. First, we need **historical imagination**; this enables us to see how the world has changed and to understand the past world that we have lost. This shows us how that lost world was better and worse, similar and different from the present. This can enable us to see the present more critically, not just as the outcome of inevitable 'progress'. Thus, in this book, particularly when looking at healthcare institutions, we consider the historical developments that have brought us to our present-day system with its benefits as well as its many flaws.

Second, Giddens (1986) says we should exercise an **anthropological imagination**. There have been (and to some extent still are) many types of societies and cultures throughout the world which have been organised very differently from our own. These societies often have different ideas and beliefs about nature, the body, health and illness. For example, some of these other cultures are indigenous or 'First Nation' cultures with very different ways of living. They also have practical skills and knowledge from which we can learn. We should not fall into the trap of thinking that the industrial capitalist world that we live in is the most 'developed' form of society or the pinnacle of human evolution. It is, after all, well on its way to destroying our planet. This highlights the need to learn about other cultures' values and practices, such as their knowledge of and respect for the natural world. We can use this knowledge to look more critically at our own culture and ways of living (Barkham, 2010). Sadly, many of these indigenous cultures are now threatened by discrimination, industrialisation, habitat destruction and climate change (Baird, 2008).

However, according to Giddens, there is always the possibility of change. The third way that we can exercise the sociological imagination is through a **critique of existing social arrangements** and forms of society. Unlike the natural and physical sciences, the subject matter of sociology is not governed by unalterable laws. Comparisons with the past and with other cultures can help us to gain some necessary critical distance from our own and allow us to reimagine a better future. Critiques leading to change can happen both at a 'micro' level, such as how a ward is organised, or at a 'macro' level, such as tackling racial inequalities in health. Giddens thus says that we need to develop our critical faculties to imagine and effect change for the better, and sociology can help us to achieve this. Similarly, Bauman (2015) says that sociology is the 'science of freedom'. It challenges the belief that 'things just are the way they are' and cannot be changed. Bauman and May (2019) also say that sociology has an 'antifixating' power which shows us new possibilities:

It renders flexible again the world hitherto oppressive in its apparent fixity; it shows it as a world which could be different to what it is now.

(BAUMAN & MAY, 2019, p. 16)

As health professionals, we work in institutions that have power over people, and these are people who are often vulnerable and dependent on our care. As we will see throughout the book, there are structural inequalities that affect who gets sick and how people are treated once they become sick. We can reinforce those inequalities, for example, by perpetuating ageist stereotypes in respect of our older patients (see Chapter 10), or we can challenge them. According to Goffman (1983), sociologists should pay particular attention to the exercise of institutional authority, and sociology's 'warrant' should be to carry out independent investigations into those people and institutions who exercise power over others. He says:

If one must have warrant addressed to social needs, let it be for unsponsored analyses of the social arrangements enjoyed by those with institutional authority-priests, psychiatrists, school teachers, police, generals, government leaders, parents, males, whites, nationals, media operators, and all the other well-placed persons who are in a position to give official imprint to versions of reality.

(GOFFMAN, 1983, p. 17)

Goffman believed we needed to question 'official' versions of reality. His study of 'total institutions', which we discuss in Chapter 10, addressed this 'warrant'. We will also discuss his analysis of stigma in relation to poverty, obesity, disability and long-term illness. Throughout this book, we will take a critical look at how institutions and their staff exercise power over others. We will also consider how these institutions reproduce social inequalities. This will lead us to look at concepts such as class prejudice, institutional racism, sexism, ageism, stigma, victim blaming and disability discrimination.

Next, we will consider how sociologists work and how they exercise the sociological imagination through the production of sociological theories and evidence.

How Sociologists Work

Giddens (2015) suggests that sociology involves a **scientific approach** to social life, but he argues that sociologists have a conception of science that is different from that employed in the natural sciences. Sociologists strive to investigate social life with rigour and impartiality but have a wider view of what constitutes evidence. The matters that sociologists investigate are complex, so sociologists rarely find experimental methods useful, since they depend on isolating a single variable from its context. Understanding context is central to sociological work. Instead, sociologists make use of a wide range of quantitative and qualitative methods, such as the social survey, interviewing, secondary analysis of official data, ethnography, case study and historical research. They also place emphasis on theory development and understanding the relationship between evidence and theory. **Sociological theories** give logical abstract explanations of social phenomena which help us to understand social reality.

Another important thing to say about how sociologists work is that sociological knowledge is reflexive. Sociologists therefore see reflexivity as central to the rigour of sociological work. **Reflexivity** refers to the critical examination of one's own beliefs, assumptions and research practices. In particular, it involves considering how our own social position affects how we see the world and other people. Sociology studies human beings who have consciousness and also self-consciousness. Thus sociologists acknowledge that the subjects of a sociological inquiry are capable of reflecting on that inquiry in ways that can change both their perceptions and their behaviour. Sociologists must therefore learn to reflect critically on both the impact of their work on their research participants and the influence of their own social position and preconceptions on their work (Ransome, 2010).

Sociologists also study society at different **levels.** Sociology at the **'micro'** level looks at the behaviours and experiences of individuals or social interaction within small groups. **'Meso'** level analysis looks at how institutions, groups or networks, such as a hospital, are organised and function. **'Macro'** sociology looks at wider structures in society, for example, by looking at inequalities related to social class, gender or ethnicity.

Some Key Sociological Ideas

Sociology has a distinctive view of what constitutes **society,** seeing it as more than the sum of its parts. In other words, society is not just a collection of individuals acting independently. In this respect, sociology is engaged in an argument against individualism. We are all made, sustained and constrained by the societies, social groups and social institutions that make up the world we inhabit. Sociology concurs with the words of the Elizabethan poet, John Donne (which apply equally to women, etc.):

No man is an island; entire of itself, every man is a piece of the continent, a part of the main.

(DONNE, 1998)

Society is expressed not just in large-scale institutions such as parliament or the NHS. It is also expressed in our intimate everyday habits and behaviours and our most personal thoughts. For example, our understandings and beliefs about our bodies and our bodily habits reflect centuries of cultural change, as we shall see in Chapter 5.

The classical sociologist, Emile Durkheim, said that it was possible to discover **'social facts'**. By this he meant that there were discoverable patterns in society that reflected social 'forces' external to individuals but having an influence over their lives, their consciousness and their actions. He describes social facts as the collective beliefs and tendencies of a social group (Durkheim, 2023). The example that he used to explain this was variations in patterns of suicide. For example, he noted higher rates of suicide among Protestants than among Catholics. He suggested that this was due to stronger social solidarity and control over personal behaviour in Catholic societies (Durkheim, 2005). The meaning of his findings has since been much debated, but he was one of the first to establish that there were aggregated patterns in society that could be seen as reflecting social structures.

Emile Durkheim (1858–1917) was a French sociologist who is seen as one of the founders of the discipline alongside Karl Marx and Max Weber (see Chapter 2). Durkheim was particularly interested in how social stability and order were maintained over time, how culture was transmitted from one generation to the next, and how societies were held together by collective rituals and beliefs that reinforced reciprocal social relationships. He coined the term 'collective consciousness' to describe the shared ideas, beliefs and values of a social group. He also pioneered the use of quantitative methods in sociology. He is seen as a structural sociologist who influenced the creation of the functionalist perspective in sociology (see Chapter 6). He was also one of the first writers on professionalism (see Chapter 9).

One of the core debates in sociology is about the relationship between these social 'structures' and social action. **Structure** refers to fixed social relations in society that constrain people's actions (or opportunities for action), such as inequalities of class, race or gender. When we talk about **action**, we also talk about **agency**, which refers to an individual's ability to act independently of social influences, social constraints and social pressures. Some sociologists focus more on social structures and how they constrain people's lives, while others pay more attention to 'agency' by studying people's everyday actions and interactions with others. We may, of course, consider that both are important parts of a sociological understanding of the world and that while our actions can change the world around us to some degree, they are also constrained by structural forces over which we have little control.

Another core debate is about whether sociologists focus attention on societal **consensus** or societal **conflict**. We discuss the ideas of the 'functionalist' sociologist, Talcott Parsons, in Chapter 6. Parsons' theories about what he called 'the social system' suggested that society was built on shared norms and values. Thus he emphasised the importance of maintaining social cohesion, equilibrium and consensus. Critics have argued that he ignored the existence of social inequality and social conflict and uncritically accepted the status quo. Critical theorists, by contrast, focus more on understanding inequality, social injustice and conflict in society. An example is the conflict theorist C. Wright Mills, discussed earlier. Critical theorists thus often focus more on social reform than social stability (Ransome, 2010). Throughout this book we consider a variety of sociological theories and theorists who have taken varying positions on these two debates. These theorists and their theories will be introduced and explained as they come up. We will also draw on a variety of different types of empirical evidence including both research evidence and some illustrative case examples.

Another key concept in sociology is that of **culture,** and Durkheim was the first sociologist to pay detailed attention to culture. There is no single definition of culture. Culture is often described as the 'way of life' of a social group. Giddens and Sutton (2017) describe culture as:

> *The values, norms, habits and ways of life characteristic of a coherent social group.*

(p. 994)

We consider many cultural issues throughout this book. For example, we consider how the culture of colonialism led to racism in Chapter 4. We consider cultural ideas about the body and illness in Chapters 5 and 6. We also consider the culture of organisations in Chapters 8–10. Here we consider the cultural dominance of particular political ideas such as neoliberalism and managerialism, and in Chapter 9, we use the concept of 'McDonaldisation' to illustrate the impact of these ideas on healthcare.

Ideas About Health and Illness

The sociology of health and illness considers the impact of society and culture on the preservation of health, the development of illness and the experience of illness. It also considers healthcare systems as social institutions. In this section we will consider how the sociological understanding of health and illness fits alongside other ways of thinking about illness.

We can contrast the sociological approach to illness with the biomedical model of illness. We look at the **biomedical model** of illness in more detail in Chapter 6. Briefly, we can characterise the biomedical model as a model that seeks the cause of illness within the patient's body. Key characteristics of the biomedical model are that it is **individualistic** in that it looks at the individual patient in isolation from their social and environmental context. It is also **reductionist**, by which we mean that it reduces all symptoms, problems and difficulties (e.g. pain or anxiety) to the physical structure and functions of the human body (Nettleton, 2020). Biomedicine is often unwilling to acknowledge the contextual factors which influence health, treating them as irrelevant 'noise' which should be ignored. We look at this in more detail in Chapter 6 when we discuss diagnosis.

There are branches of medicine which move beyond a narrow biomedical model of illness. **Public health** medicine is concerned with the health of the population and in particular with protecting and promoting population health. It is underpinned by the discipline of **epidemiology**, which studies the distribution, spread and control of disease. Epidemiologists study how many people have a disease and how that disease is spreading, and they also consider the factors that have affected the spread of a disease. One of the key features of epidemiological research is the use of comparisons to identify factors causing disease, for example, comparing rates of lung cancer in smokers and non-smokers (Coggon et al., 2009). Epidemiology has therefore made a very valuable contribution to our knowledge of what are called the 'social determinants' of health (see below).

However, epidemiology tends to be focused on the causes of disease rather than taking a wider view of what we might describe as the **'causes of the causes'** (Braveman and Gottlieb, 2014). For example, epidemiology might find an association between poverty and ill health but tends not to explore the causes of poverty. There are areas of convergence between epidemiology and the sociology of health and illness but also areas of divergence. Sociology pays more attention to the social 'causes of causes' of ill health. In addition, while epidemiology focuses exclusively on disease aetiology (meaning the cause of disease), sociology of health and illness covers other issues as well, such as people's experiences of illness and treatment. Sociologists also investigate the social organisation of healthcare institutions and health work. Despite their differences, in many ways, the two disciplines complement each other.

We have said that public health is concerned with protecting the health of populations, and it does this through the control and regulation of disease. According to Omran (1971), the more affluent industrialised societies have passed through an **'epidemiological transition'** in which there have been changing patterns of mortality, life expectancy, fertility and causes of death. In brief, people are living longer, fewer babies are being born and thus the age structure of populations has changed. The causes of death have also changed with a sharp decline in infectious diseases but increased prevalence of what Omran described as degenerative and man-made diseases. Although subsequent authors have critiqued Omran's theory as an overgeneralisation, it has been influential in shaping public health policy (Mackenbach, 2022). Thus, while earlier public health approaches were concerned with controlling the spread of infectious diseases, a central concern of contemporary public health (particularly in the affluent West) has been the control and management of non-communicable diseases such as cardiovascular disease, diabetes and cancer. This is one reason that public health bodies in more affluent Western countries were so often unprepared for the COVID-19 pandemic.

Contemporary public health approaches to non-communicable disease, while drawing on an understanding of social determinants of health, tend to look to individualised solutions, with the central focus of much public health discourse in the UK being on individual **'lifestyle factors'** such as diet and exercise. This is partly due to the centrality of the idea of risk in much public health discourse. **Risk** is defined in terms of the probability of an individual within a specific population developing a health problem (Coggon et al., 2009). Public health (and medicine in general) has increasingly moved towards a 'population health' approach focused on the management of risk. First, this involves the surveillance of the health of populations through surveys and routine data collection to establish the existence of health problems such as obesity at a population level. Second, it involves intervening to address these problems.

In the UK and many other affluent Western countries, interventions are mainly focused on individuals. Often these interventions involve the assessment of individuals and their 'risk factors' with a view to implementing **'health promotion'** activities such as weight loss advice to modify these risks. This type of approach tends to be limited in its attempts to address the 'causes of the causes' such as the promotion of ultra-processed foods that are high in fat, salt and sugar by the food industry. Armstrong (1995), following the ideas of Michel Foucault (see Chapter 5), has suggested that medicine is moving away from the biomedical model towards a new model that he calls **'surveillance medicine'**. This model is more concerned with the governance of whole populations and their health behaviours and less with the care and treatment of the sick individual. Thus Armstrong suggests that 'surveillance medicine' is more focused on managing populations than providing services for them. Surveillance medicine **'responsibilises'** sick people by transferring responsibility for their treatment and care from the health service to the individuals themselves. Thus it expects patients to, as far as possible, manage their own health problems and try to solve these problems independently of help (Peeters, 2019). This is problematic when a patient lacks the resources to do so or when a patient's problems are due to forces beyond their control (we discuss self-management in Chapter 7). We look at Armstrong's ideas in a little more detail in Chapter 10 when we look at the changing role of the hospital.

The World Health Organization describes health promotion as 'the process of enabling people to increase control over, and improve their health' (WHO, n.d.). This focus within public health and health promotion on individual behaviour change can be linked to the prevailing political culture of **'neoliberalism'** in the UK and other affluent Western countries such as the United States. We discuss neoliberalism in more depth in Chapters 8–10, but we can briefly define it as a political philosophy which seeks to promote market capitalism, reduce regulation of private enterprise, and reduce the size of the state and state services. It is also underpinned by a philosophy of individualism (Steger & Roy, 2010). Thus, in most areas of public policy, it tends to advocate individualist solutions, such as exhorting individuals to recycle more and drive less in response to climate change. This neoliberal approach is often reluctant to deliver the structural changes needed to address social problems, such as, in the case of climate change, stopping the production of fossil fuels. It has been suggested that this political reluctance to consider structural intervention underpinned the government's initial reluctance to act during the COVID-19 pandemic (Bourgeron, 2022).

We see this neoliberal approach translated into the public health field in the policy focus on '**behaviour change**'. '**Behaviour change**' programmes use behaviourist techniques to try to modify individual lifestyles, but at the same time they ignore structural determinants of illness such as inequality and environmental degradation (Ratcliff, 2017). Behaviour change programmes enact the idea of '**responsibilisation**'. They promote the idea that individuals must be trained into taking responsibility for their health, and for the management of any sickness or disability that afflicts them (Peeters, 2019). This has been called 'victim blaming'.

VICTIM BLAMING

Crawford (1977) described '**victim blaming**' as an ideology which blames the individual for their illness. He suggested that this ideology was employed to justify cuts in health and welfare services by blaming the sick for engaging in 'faulty' habits and 'risky' behaviours. He says that this ideology diverts attention away from the social, commercial and industrial causes of disease.

Victim blaming has created a moralising public health discourse which blames those considered to be 'failing' to engage in 'good' health behaviours while tending to ignore those health-damaging social determinants that are beyond the individual's control. We will consider these arguments in more detail at various points in the book, particularly in Chapters 2 and 6. We will look at the social determinants of health in more detail in the next section.

Social Determinants of Health

The term '**social determinants**' of health has been defined by the World Health Organization as:

> …*the circumstances, in which people are born, grow up, live, work and age, and the systems put in place to deal with illness. These circumstances are in turn shaped by a wider set of forces: economics, social policies, and politics.*
>
> (WHO, 2013)

Much of the work that has been carried out on the social determinants of health has identified avoidable inequalities in health. These avoidable inequalities can lead to avoidable illness, disability and death. We tackle these inequalities in depth in Chapters 2–4. The WHO has identified a range of social determinants which are implicated in health inequalities and avoidable harm to health. These include:

> *Income, education, housing conditions, environmental conditions, working conditions, food insecurity, unemployment, access to basic amenities such as clean water and heating, access to transport, social inclusion/exclusion and access to healthcare and support for early childhood development.*
>
> (WHO, 2008)

Subsequent to the WHO report, other researchers have added new social determinants to this list, with a particular focus on identifying the 'causes of the causes' of health inequalities (Braveman and Gottlieb, 2014). For example, a number of authors have researched the concept of '**corporate and commercial determinants**' of ill health. In an era of globalization, these can be difficult for individual governments to control. A review by Mialon (2020) identified three types of commercial determinants of ill health. First, corporations promote harmful products such as fast foods and tobacco. Second, they use health-damaging business practices such as providing poor working conditions and insecure, badly paid jobs; damaging the environment; evading taxes; and engaging in political lobbying to block health interventions which might affect their profits, such as controls on gambling and alcohol consumption (Hastings, 2012). Finally, Mialon says that corporations are 'global drivers' of ill health. Globalisation has given enormous power to transnational corporations, which they have used to shape political and economic conditions that are favourable to their interests. For example, they have opposed the regulation of harmful products and harmful business practices at an international level through their influence on international trade agreements and bodies such as the World Trade Organization. This can tie the hands of national governments that are trying to introduce public health measures.

Other authors have argued for the existence of **'political determinants'** of health, arguing that power relations, structures of power and policy decisions can create adverse social conditions for the powerless. A good example would be the Grenfell Tower fire. This caused 79 deaths and was preventable. The Grenfell residents had been raising concerns about fire safety for years but were ignored, so we can trace the roots of this disaster back to the fact that residents were voiceless and powerless to change their fate (McKee, 2017). Next, we will look at a case example which brings together all these ideas to show the complex causality involved in social determinants of health.

Case Example: A Leptospirosis Outbreak

Birnbaum (2022) describes an outbreak of an infectious disease in the South Bronx neighbourhood of New York City and then explores the different social forces which contributed to the outbreak. She uses what she calls multiple 'lenses' (ways of looking) to examine the problem. The disease was leptospirosis (Weil's disease) which is a bacterial infection often spread through rat urine. It can be fatal. The initial public health response was to start in close proximity to the problem: first by setting rat traps and then by 'responsibilising' individual tenants by focusing on their hygiene practices such as hand washing. Birnbaum suggests that we next need to move to a slightly more distant 'lens' and look at the practices of landlords which led to the rat infestation. The landlord in question had habitually violated housing laws both by failing to maintain his properties and by illegally subdividing flats into smaller multioccupancy units. These conditions allowed the rat infestation to spread rapidly. Moving to a slightly wider lens again, Birnbaum looked at the housing market in New York to see why this was allowed to happen. She described marked inequalities between rich and poor neighbourhoods in New York. Low-income neighbourhoods were poorly provided with services and contained people who were 'rent burdened', spending a high proportion of their income on rent. Birnbaum said that, in these areas, landlords knew that tenants had little chance of finding somewhere else to live so would have no choice but to put up with bad conditions. Thus landlords knew they could get away with cutting back on property maintenance and illegally subdividing flats to maximise profits.

Moving to an even wider political 'lens', this situation was allowed to arise through political and policy neglect of urban decay and housing shortages alongside deregulation of the housing market which reduced controls on bad landlords. This reduced the rights of tenants, increased overcrowding and allowed landlords to neglect their properties with impunity. Moving out again to a much wider lens, we can start to put these problems into a global context. Birnbaum does this by describing an increase in what she calls 'financialisation'. This refers to the increased global dominance of financial institutions such as banks, hedge funds and private equity firms and their focus on making money through financial speculation rather than through producing goods and services. In New York, this led to large amounts of property being used for financial speculation. Lots of properties were bought up by offshore companies, some tied to international elites such as Russian oligarchs. These properties were treated simply as financial assets and left empty for much of the time. This created a severe housing shortage. This property speculation played a very important role in the New York housing crisis and thus, ultimately, in the rat infestation and leptospirosis outbreak.

Though we have travelled a long way from rats in the basement of a tenement in the South Bronx, Birnbaum is asking us to look at how all the pieces in this puzzle fit together. This was a problem that could only be fixed temporarily at an individual or local level. It will happen again and again unless some of the wider forces driving the problem are tackled. This case is a good example of why we need to engage in what is called 'upstream thinking' about the social determinants of health.

THE NEED FOR UPSTREAM THINKING

The idea of upstream thinking originates from a paper by the medical sociologist John McKinlay, first published in 1975. He told this story about a physician:

> *I am standing by the shore of a swiftly flowing river and I hear the cry of a drowning man. So I jump into the river, put my arms around him, pull him to shore and apply artificial respiration. Just when he begins to breathe, there is another cry for help. So I jump into the river, reach him, pull him to shore, apply artificial respiration, and then just as he begins to breathe, another cry for help. So back in the river … Again and again, without end, goes the sequence. You know, I am so busy jumping in, pulling them to shore … that I have no time to see who the hell is upstream pushing them all in.*

(MCKINLAY, 2019, p. 1)

McKinlay says that we all need to be educated about the wider causes of illness. At the moment, he says, there is too much 'downstream' education which lectures us about what we 'ought' and 'ought not' do; such as what we should eat; how many steps we should take in a day. Like Crawford, he calls this 'blaming the victim'. He is particularly concerned with the 'corporate determinants' of ill health, and he urges us to become more aware of the activities of the 'manufacturers of illness' who, for example, pollute our air and waterways and sell us unhealthy products. He also says that as health professionals, we need to move away from victim-blaming approaches that focus on the 'culpability' of sick individuals. He says that it was legislative interventions, such as tobacco duty and restrictions on tobacco sales and smoking in public places, that drove down smoking rates, not just telling smokers they should stop. McKinlay says that thinking 'upstream' should help us to challenge this culture of victim blaming and will give us more effective solutions to public health issues.

REFLECTION POINT

Think of some common preventable health problems, such as obesity, anxiety or back pain. Choose one health problem and suggest some 'upstream' solutions to prevent it.

Outline of the Three Sections of the Book

The book takes seriously Goffman's 'warrant' for sociology outlined earlier. It thus pays particular attention to critically examining those situations in healthcare where people and institutions exercise power over others. It also critically examines 'official' versions of reality, particularly in the final section on the organisation of health services.

Part 1: Inequality and Social Determinants of Health

The first part of the book introduces social determinants of health and examines inequalities of social class, gender and ethnicity. Key sociological theorists who are introduced include Emile

Durkheim, Karl Marx, Max Weber and Pierre Bourdieu, along with their theories. The theoretical perspective of social constructionism is introduced. Key concepts that are discussed include social class, social exclusion, the 'gender order', everyday sexism, feminism, victim blaming, 'medical gaslighting', intersectionality, institutional racism and 'othering'.

Part 2: Health and Illness as Social and Cultural Experiences

The second part of the book covers cultural perceptions of the body, the experience of illness and long-term illness and disability. Key theorists who are introduced include Michel Foucault, Erving Goffman and Talcott Parsons, alongside their theories. The sociological perspectives of phenomenology, symbolic interactionism, critical theory and functionalism are introduced. Key concepts that are discussed include the 'civilising process', 'normalising judgment', medicalisation, illness narratives, stigma, labelling, biographical disruption and the social model of disability.

Part 3: The Social and Political Organisation of Healthcare

The final part of the book covers health policy, the organisation of healthcare, professionalism and managerialism, the nature of nursing work and places of care. Key concepts that are discussed include professionalism, managerialism, neoliberalism, new public management, McDonaldisation, total institutions, governmentality, ageism, emotional labour, 'dirty' work and the 'corruption' of care.

Further Reading

Bauman, Z., & May, T. (2019). *Thinking sociologically.* John Wiley & Sons.
McKinlay, J. B. (2019). A case for refocusing upstream: The political economy of illness. *IAPHS Occasional Classics, 1*, 1–10.
Mills, C. W. (2000). *The sociological imagination.* Oxford University Press.

References

Armstrong, D. (1995). The rise of surveillance medicine. *Sociology of Health & Illness, 17*(3), 393–404.
Baird, R. (2008). *The impact of climate change on minorities and indigenous peoples.* Minority Rights Group International.
Barkham, P. (2010). Save the planet—A message from another world. *The Guardian.* Retrieved January 2, 2024, from. https://www.theguardian.com/environment/2010/sep/27/kogi-warn-the-west.
Bauman, Z. (2015). Sociology as a science/technology of freedom. In K. Twamley, M. Doidge, & A. Scott (Eds.), *Sociologists' tales: Contemporary narratives on sociological thought and practice* (pp. 29–34). Policy Press.
Bauman, Z., & May, T. (2019). *Thinking sociologically.* John Wiley & Sons.
Bourgeron, T. (2022). 'Let the virus spread'. A doctrine of pandemic management for the libertarian-authoritarian capital accumulation regime. *Organization, 29*(3), 401–413.
Braveman, P., & Gottlieb, L. (2014). The social determinants of health: It's time to consider the causes of the causes. *Public Health Reports, 129*(Suppl 2), 19–31.
Coggon, D., Barker, D., & Rose, G. (2009). *Epidemiology for the uninitiated.* John Wiley & Sons.
Crawford, R. (1977). You are dangerous to your health: The ideology and politics of victim blaming. *International Journal of Health Services, 7*(4), 663–680.
Donne, J. (1998). *Selected poetry.* Oxford University Press.
Durkheim, E. (2005). *Suicide: A study in sociology.* Routledge.
Durkheim, E. (2023). The rules of sociological method. In W. Longhofer, & D. Winchester (Eds.), *Social theory re-wired: New connections to classical and contemporary perspectives* (pp. 9–14). Routledge.
Giddens, A. (1986). *Sociology: A brief but critical introduction.* Bloomsbury Publishing.
Giddens, A. (2015). Why sociology matters. In K. Twamley, M. Doidge, & A. Scott (Eds.), *Sociologists' tales: Contemporary narratives on sociological thought and practice* (pp. 35–40). Policy Press.
Giddens, A., & Sutton, P. (2017). *Sociology.* Polity Press.
Goffman, E. (1983). The interaction order: American Sociological Association, 1982 presidential address. *American Sociological Review, 48*(1), 1–17.

Harmer, A., Eder, B., Gepp, S., Leetz, A., & Van de Pas, R. (2020). WHO should declare climate change a public health emergency. *BMJ, 368*, m797.

Hastings, G. (2012). Why corporate power is a public health priority. *BMJ, 345*, e5124.

Mackenbach, J. P. (2022). Omran's 'epidemiologic transition' 50 years on. *International Journal of Epidemiology, 51*(4), 1054–1057.

McKee, M. (2017). Grenfell Tower fire: Why we cannot ignore the political determinants of health. *BMJ, 357*, j2966.

McKinlay, J. B. (2019). A case for refocusing upstream: The political economy of illness. *IAPHS Occasional Classics, 1*, 1–10.

Mialon, M. (2020). An overview of the commercial determinants of health. *Globalization and Health, 16*, 1–7.

Mills, C. W. (2000). *The sociological imagination*. Oxford University Press.

Nettleton, S. (2020). *The sociology of health and illness*. John Wiley & Sons.

Omran, A. R. (1971). The epidemiologic transition: A theory of the epidemiology of population change. *Milbank Memorial Fund Quarterly, 49*, 509–538.

Peeters, R. (2019). Manufacturing responsibility: The governmentality of behavioural power in social policies. *Social Policy and Society, 18*(1), 51–65.

Prasad, A. (2022). Anti-science misinformation and conspiracies: COVID-19, post-truth, and science & technology studies (STS). *Science, Technology and Society, 27*(1), 88–112.

Ransome, P. (2010). *Social theory for beginners*. Policy Press.

Ratcliff, K. S. (2017). *The social determinants of health: Looking upstream*. John Wiley & Sons.

Solomon, C. G., & LaRocque, R. C. (2019). Climate change—A health emergency. *New England Journal of Medicine, 380*(3), 209–211.

Steger, M. B., & Roy, R. K. (2010). *Neoliberalism: A very short introduction*. Oxford University Press.

Traynor, M. (2018). Guest editorial: What's wrong with resilience? *Journal of Research in Nursing, 23*(1), 5–8.

Webster, C. (2002). *The national health service: A political history*. Oxford University Press.

World Health Organization (WHO). (2008). *Closing the gap in a generation: Health equity through action on the social determinants of health: Commission on social determinants of health final report*. Retrieved January 2, 2024, from. https://www.who.int/publications/i/item/WHO-IER-CSDH-08.1.

World Health Organization (WHO). (2013). *Social determinants of health: Key concepts*. Retrieved January 2, 2024, from. https://www.who.int/news-room/questions-and-answers/item/social-determinants-of-health-key-concepts.

World Health Organization (WHO). (n.d.). *Health promotion*. Retrieved January 2, 2024, from https://www.who.int/westernpacific/about/how-we-work/programmes/health-promotion.

Social Class and Inequalities of Health

In the first chapter, you were introduced to the concept of 'social determinants' of health. This concept suggests that social conditions can increase the risk of individuals becoming sick and dying prematurely. This chapter looks at social class as a social determinant of health. There is no greater inequality than dying earlier because you are poorer. However, we know that being less well-off can shorten your life expectancy and increase your chances of suffering from long-term illness. We call these inequalities in health and wellbeing the 'social gradient', since they affect not just the richest and poorest but all levels of society. Thus even people in the middle ranks of society have a lower life expectancy than those better off than them. In this chapter, we will be looking at what this means, the evidence for the existence of a social gradient in life expectancy, and its negative effect on the health of populations.

What Is Social Class?

SOCIOLOGICAL IDEAS ABOUT CLASS

We use the term *social class* to group together people who have similar amounts of resources, such as money and property. People from a particular class share similar levels of income, wealth and life chances, and these are frequently passed down from one generation to the next (Giddens, 2021). Thus, when we talk about social class, we are suggesting that society is not just a collection of individuals with different abilities, jobs and lifestyle preferences. Instead, we can see regular patterns in society which shape and constrain individual life chances. For example, only 7% of the population is privately educated, but in 2019, former private school pupils made up 67% of judges, 59% of senior civil servants, 44% of newspaper columnists and 29% of Members of Parliament (MPs) (Hecht et al., 2020).

Karl Marx: Political Economy and Class

Karl Marx (1818–1883) was a political economist, historian and sociologist who is best known for his work, 'The Communist Manifesto', written with Friedrich Engels in Manchester in 1848. As a result of this work, he is often seen as a political activist rather than an academic; however, the communist regimes founded in places like Russia and China bore little similarity to Marx's original ideas. Most of Marx's life was devoted to philosophical and political analysis of the Industrial Revolution and the growth of capitalism, particularly in his major work, 'Capital'. Marx believed that societal change was driven by class conflict, and his work has been influential among theorists studying conflict and social inequalities. One of the key concepts he developed was 'alienation', which described a sense of estrangement and worthlessness felt by workers who no longer felt they had any control over their lives, work or destiny. His work has been used to understand the economic roots of health inequalities.

Marx was one of the first people to define social class. He thought that class was ultimately about the ownership of land and property. Marx said that the 'ownership of the means of production' by, for example, mill and factory owners allowed them to control their workers' lives and extract profits from their labour. He called this capital-owning class the 'bourgeoisie'. This exploitation could impoverish workers while allowing the bourgeoisie to become extremely wealthy (Marx, 2016).

Marx's ideas were important in demonstrating the key role of economic exploitation in driving inequality and poverty. He suggested that it is mainly labour which creates wealth, yet that wealth is expropriated as profit by the 'bourgeoisie'. He also suggested that it is in the interests of the bourgeoisie to drive down the wages of their workers to increase profits, and over time this leads to the 'immiseration' (increased misery) of working people, leading to class conflict. However, the class system developed a level of complexity through the 20th century which he did not predict, particularly through the growth of managerial and professional members of the middle class. Class conflict was also tempered by the successes of the trade union movement in improving working conditions as well as the creation of welfare states. However, some of these developments have been reversed since the 1980s, and some recent authors have built on Marx's ideas to explain worsening inequalities in the 21st century (Piketty, 2014). Although Marx's ideas have remained influential, contemporary understandings of social class, particularly those used in official measures of class, have often been influenced by the ideas of a later classical sociologist called Max Weber.

Max Weber: Class, Status and Power

Max Weber (1864–1920) was a German sociologist who analysed key social changes in industrial capitalist societies. He was concerned with the growth of bureaucracy, rationalisation and secularisation in modern societies. He is particularly known for his work, 'The Protestant Ethic and the Spirit of Capitalism', which looked at the impact of Protestant theology on the development of capitalism. His analysis of bureaucracy and the growth of 'calculative rationality' in modern society has been important to the study of organisations. Weber also pioneered a sociological concern with the subjective meaning of social phenomena. He called this 'Verstehen' (meaning interpretive understanding), and the concept has been important to the development of qualitative research methods. His ideas underpin the official measure of class in the UK. His ideas about bureaucracy have been used to understand healthcare organisations.

Weber built upon Marx's ideas but thought that there was more to social class than Marx's basic distinction between the owners of the means of production and the 'wage slaves' who were forced to sell them their labour. Weber identified three key attributes of social class, which he called class, status and party (Gerth & Mills, 2014).

Weber agreed with Marx that the ownership of wealth was an important determinant of class position. However, Weber thought that factors such as status also had importance. For example, some occupations, such as clergy, artists and writers, could have the benefits of cultural status and respect despite lacking wealth. He also thought that the amount of political power and control that people could exercise was important. He called this 'party'. So we can sum up Weber's argument by saying that social class is about three things: (1) how much wealth and income you have, (2) how much prestige or status you have and (3) how much power and autonomy you have. Weber also suggested that an individual's 'market position' affected their social class. Factors such as skills and qualifications could allow people to ascend to a higher position in the class structure (Giddens, 2021). However, it is important to remember that the social background and wealth of your family can affect your access to these skills and qualifications. We noted this earlier when we discussed the privileged access to elite positions afforded to former private school pupils.

Pierre Bourdieu: Social and Cultural Capital

Pierre Bourdieu (1930–2002) was a French sociologist, mainly known as a sociologist of education and culture. He was concerned with how social hierarchies were perpetuated. He partly built on the ideas of Marx and Durkheim but criticised the idea that inequality was purely reproduced through economic factors. He introduced the concepts of social and cultural capital to explain how privilege was culturally reproduced. He also introduced the concept of symbolic violence to explain non-physical forms of violence which are imposed on subordinate groups in society to maintain the status quo; for example, by denigrating the worth of the disadvantaged. He thought that the disadvantaged could internalise this symbolic violence, leading to feelings of low self-worth. His work has been used in the sociology of health to understand how inequalities of health are culturally reproduced.

Bourdieu partly drew on the ideas of Marx to look at how people from different class backgrounds have differential access, not only to economic resources but also to social and cultural resources. People can thus use a combination of economic, cultural and social resources to obtain advantages and privileges for themselves and pass these down through their families. For example, looking at education, he noticed how the middle and upper classes had cultural advantages in both the education system and the workplace, and he called these advantages **'cultural capital'**. He described cultural capital as 'fluency' in the culture of the elite, that is, having the required mannerisms, vocabulary, accent, cultural tastes and dress to demonstrate that you belong in a particular class. This can then allow you to demonstrate that you 'belong' in a particular social space, such as an elite university. Demonstrating that you 'belong' can be demonstrated by the consumption of 'right' high-status cultural products such as art, music, books and travel (Bourdieu, 1984). For example, middle-class parents may pay for extracurricular classes or gap year experiences that they believe will give their children the 'edge' when applying to elite universities (Heath, 2007).

Bourdieu also showed how the more affluent classes had access to social contacts, which gave them and their children advantages that people from poorer backgrounds did not have. He called this privileged access **'social capital'**. We have already considered how private education can give people access to high-status jobs. Another good example would be the way in which access to prestigious jobs is often linked to unpaid internships. Access to these may be limited and they are often filled through word-of-mouth contacts (Hecht et al., 2020). The acquisition of social and cultural capital is therefore often closely linked to the possession of economic capital. Thus gaining the experience, skills and qualifications that, in Weber's terms, give you a good 'market position' may depend not only on your family's social contacts but also on the 'bank of mum and dad' (Toft & Friedman, 2020).

HOW WE MEASURE SOCIAL CLASS IN THE UK

We have known for many years, from research studies, that social class has both positive and negative impacts on many aspects of people's lives, including their health and life expectancy. In order to assess its impact, it is important that we have an agreed measure of social class and many countries have similar official measures. In this country, we now use a measure called the National Statistics Socio-economic Classification of Classes (NS-SEC). This classifies occupations according to pay, status and other factors such as job security and autonomy, drawing on Weber's original ideas. The NS-SEC classification identifies eight classes, which run from class 1 which includes higher professional and management jobs to class 7 which includes people in routine jobs such as manual labour or working behind a bar. The unemployed and other people on benefits, such as people with disabilities, are classified separately as class 8. Students are also classified separately (Office for National Statistics, 2010) (Table 2.1).

Changes in the Class Structure

INDUSTRIAL DECLINE

When Marx was writing about class, the economy of the UK was dependent on industrial manufacturing, and large sections of the population worked in manufacturing industries such as steel and textile production. There were very clear distinctions between the classes in terms of how they dressed, how they spoke, and so on. The working classes were largely employed in manual labour jobs, working in places such as mines and factories. People in these industries had a strong sense of belonging, sometimes described as **class consciousness**. Since the 1960s, manufacturing industries have declined dramatically in the UK. In 1948, manufacturing made up 41% of the economy, but by 2015, this had fallen to 14% (ONS, 2014). We now import most of our manufactured goods from places like China. As a result, the service sector now comprises 79% of the UK economy.

Thus most people in the UK now work in non-manual jobs in the service sector in places such as shops, bars, hotels, care homes and call centres. These are 'white collar' jobs that superficially appear to be 'middle class', yet many are routine, poorly paid and insecure, so they still share many of the

TABLE 2.1 ■ **Key Statistics and Quick Statistics for Local Authorities in the United Kingdom**

Classification	Example	Percentage of Population
1. Higher managerial, administrative and professional	Consultant surgeon, army officer, chief executive	10%
2. Lower managerial, administrative and professional	Teacher, journalist, nurse, midwife	21%
3. Intermediate	Medical secretary, travel agent, police constable	13%
4. Small employers and own account workers	Farmer, owner taxi driver, hotel manager	9%
5. Lower supervisory and technical occupations	Gardener, train driver, electrician	7%
6. Semi-routine occupations	Traffic warden, care worker, dental nurse	14%
7. Routine occupations	Building labourer, waiter, cleaner	11%
8. Never worked/long-term unemployed		6%

Based on data from Office for National Statistics (ONS). (2013). 2011 Census: Key statistics and quick statistics for local authorities in the United Kingdom. Retrieved December 12, 2023, from https://www.ons.gov.uk/employmentandlabourmarket/peopleinwork/employmentandemployeetypes/bulletins/keystatisticsand quickstatisticsforlocalauthoritiesintheunitedkingdom/2013-12-04.

characteristics of more traditional 'working class' jobs. Standing (2014) has coined the term 'precariat' to describe service workers whose work is insecure and unpredictable. Examples of precarious work include temporary work, agency work, 'zero hours' contracts and what Standing calls 'phony' self-employment. There are growing numbers of precarious jobs which share poor conditions of work such as job insecurity, high job demands, low wages and a lack of employment benefits such as sick pay and a pension. Zero hours contracts increased fivefold between 2010 and 2019 and affected 900,000 people (Marmot et al., 2020). As we will see later, these work conditions are known to be detrimental to health in similar ways to the industrial jobs of the past (Muntaner, 2018).

The decline of industry and manufacturing has brought big economic changes at a societal level that have profoundly changed the everyday lives of ordinary people. Deindustrialisation has deepened levels of inequality in the UK. However, while economic inequalities have increased, people are less certain about which class they identify with and may not feel a sense of community with people from a similar background (Silva & Warde, 2010). Savage (2015) has suggested that these economic changes have fragmented both middle- and working-class communities in this country. At the same time, the elite has 'pulled away' from the rest of the population in terms of its wealth, power and privileges (Hecht et al., 2020).

GEOGRAPHICAL INEQUALITIES

In the previous section, we looked at how the world has changed since the early studies of class in the 19th century. In the 19th and much of the 20th centuries, those working in mills or factories in industrial towns faced poor working conditions and low wages. In Great Britain, there was a distinct north-south divide, with poorer communities more heavily concentrated in manufacturing towns in northern England, South Wales and southern Scotland, while wealth was concentrated in southern England. The north has also traditionally received far less public investment, particularly in education, transport and healthcare. There are also some poor areas in the south. London, in particular, has some areas of extreme poverty, such as Tower Hamlets, while rural poverty affects areas such as the South West. Coastal towns are now also some of the poorest places in Britain (Hudson, 2013).

As British industry declined, the old industrial communities in places like northern England, South Wales and the Scottish lowlands suffered economic decline as enterprises such as coal mines, factories and steel works progressively closed down (Hudson, 2013). New secure jobs are often concentrated in more affluent parts of the country, such as London or Cambridge. This has left behind many 'post-industrial' towns and villages where work for younger people is scarce and precarious. Meanwhile, the older generation may still be suffering from the health-damaging effects of former heavy industries; for example, the respiratory diseases associated with mining, so their children may be tied to the locality by caring responsibilities (Shucksmith et al., 2010). Growing evidence has suggested that the economic changes in the UK since the 1980s have led to worsening geographical inequalities and, in particular, a deepening north-south divide. The austerity policies pursued following the 2008 financial crisis sharply accelerated these trends (Lansley & Mack, 2015).

Thus, there have been profound geographical inequalities in the UK for at least 2 centuries, but these have worsened since the 1980s, with a particularly sharp increase in inequality since the 2008 financial crisis.

How Is Inequality Growing in the UK?

INCOME INEQUALITY

We have seen that economic inequality is increasing, so now we are going to briefly consider some evidence concerning levels of inequality in the UK today. First, we need to think about UK inequality against the backdrop of staggering global inequality. For example:

- Worldwide, one person dies every 4 seconds as a result of inequality (Ahmed et al., 2022).
- The 10 richest men in the world own more than the bottom 3.1 billion people (Ahmed et al., 2022).
- The richest 1% hold 45.6% of global wealth, while the poorest 50% of the world have just 0.75% (Christensen, 2023).
- The very wealthy within a country like the UK now see themselves as part of a global elite divorced from the lives of ordinary citizens (Hecht et al., 2020).

We can think of economic inequality in two ways. First, we will consider income inequality (what you earn), and second, wealth inequality (the money, land and property that you own). Looking first at income inequality, we can see that one of the particular features of inequality in the UK is a very big difference between the income of the top 1% and the other 99%.

- In 2022, the average (median) income in the UK was £33,061. Most of the population earned less than this figure.
- Around 50,000 people in the top income bracket accounted for 6% of all earnings – 60 times greater than their population share. More than half of the top 1% richest adults lived in London and the southeast, and only one-fifth were women (Delestre et al., 2022).
- Chief executive (CEO) pay now averages over 100 times the pay of an average worker and 165 times that of an average nurse. The CEOs of the top FTSE100 companies earn, on average, £4.5 million. These pay differentials have gone up enormously since the 1970s (Equality Trust, 2021).
- These differentials are highlighted by High Pay Day. This is the day in the year when individual CEOs in top companies have already received the pay that an average UK worker will receive in a year. In 2023, this occurred at 2 pm on 5 January (High Pay Centre, 2023).

All these figures tell us that the UK is now a very unequal society and that inequality has increased dramatically since the 1980s. The UK had become a less unequal country in the period from the 1940s to the 1970s after the welfare state was created. However, this progress was reversed after 1980. As a result, the UK is now more unequal than most other European countries (Dorling, 2018).

International comparisons have shown that countries vary not only in levels of inequality but also in perceptions of inequality. There is often a mismatch between the actual level of inequality in a country and the extent to which its population understands its reality. The UK is one of a small number of developed countries where levels of inequality are high, but the public perceives levels of inequality to be much lower than they actually are. Surveys have shown that people in the UK systematically underestimate levels of income inequality. Most people have little idea just how much more money the highest paid earn compared to the average worker (Rowlingson & Mackay, 2013).

INEQUALITY OF WEALTH

So far we have looked at what people earn but we are now going to look at the wealth that people own. Here, there are even bigger differences between the richest and poorest groups in Britain, especially between the richest 1% and the other 99%.

- The richest 10% of the population own 45% of the country's wealth, while the poorest 10% own only 2% (Office for National Statistics, 2019).
- The richest 1% of the population owns 22% of the country's wealth, and this figure has increased from 15% in 1984 (World Inequality Lab, 2018).

Wealth in Britain also tends to be concentrated in the South East of England. A troubling finding is that the poorest 10% of the population own less than nothing, having debts amounting to three times their assets. These are often people in precarious employment who are forced to borrow money to pay for necessities such as utility bills. Wealth inequality in the UK is twice as high as income inequality, and we can see from these figures that there is a growing divide between the richest and poorest in society. These inequalities are also exacerbated by geographical inequalities, in particular the north-south divide. As a result of these high levels of inequality, social mobility has stalled, and it has become more difficult for people to move out of the class into which they were born (Hills et al., 2010). We will consider this issue next.

REFLECTION POINT

Some sociologists have argued that 'class consciousness' has declined in the UK. Think about what social class means to you. Do you feel that the idea of social class is a meaningful way of thinking about your position in life? Do you have a clear idea of which social class you belong to? What impact do you think that a decline in 'class consciousness' might have on tackling social inequality?

SOCIAL MOBILITY

The term **social mobility** refers to movement up or down the social hierarchy. A society with high levels of social mobility offers a lot of opportunities for individuals to achieve a higher position in society than that of their parents. Social mobility is often represented in the media through the 'rags to riches' stories of prominent individuals such as Alan Sugar, who reportedly started his career selling electrical goods from a van and is now a billionaire businessman. The prominence of these stories in the media can convince the public that Britain is an open society where anyone with skills and talent can rise to the top. We live in a culture that widely promotes the idea that we can be whatever we want if we try hard enough. As we shall see, the reality for most people may be very different.

Example: Thinking About Social Mobility

Young white guy (about 16–18 years old, fed up, stacking shelves): 'I'm sick of this job, I wanna proper job, you know where you have to wear a suit and all that and you get to tell other people what to do'.
Young black guy (similar age, laughing, stacking shelves): 'Yeah but what do your mum and dad do for a living'?
'Young white guy (stops stacking shelves for a moment): 'Me dad drives a van and me mum works in a caff'.
Young black guy (laughing): 'So what do you expect then?'

(CROMPTON, 2010, p. 1)

We saw in the previous section that Britain is a very unequal society where levels of inequality are rising (OECD, 2016). According to Giddens (2021), there were several studies of social mobility in the UK between the 1950s and the 1980s, and these showed that there was a lot of 'short-range' mobility in the UK. In other words, people moved one rung up the social ladder to a position a little higher than that of their parents. By contrast, 'long-range' mobility, or moving several rungs up the ladder, was very rare (Giddens, 2021).

More recent studies have suggested that even that limited amount of social mobility in the UK is now declining (Sutton Trust and Social Mobility Commission, 2019). According to Hills et al (2010), this is due to rising levels of inequality since the 1980s. They suggest that if the rungs of a ladder are further apart, then the ladder is harder to climb (Hills et al., 2010). Successive governments have promoted education as the best route to increased social mobility (Reay, 2013). However, improving educational opportunities for the disadvantaged has not had the hoped-for effects of increasing social mobility (Reay, 2013). International comparisons show that UK children have a higher chance of staying in the same class as their parents than children from most other developed countries (Causa & Johansson, 2009).

Crompton (2010) argues that most individuals in the UK end up doing similar jobs to their parents. She suggests that this is due to a shortage of skilled and better-paid jobs. While low-status, badly paid jobs make up a large part of the UK job market, the opportunities for people to rise up the employment ladder will remain limited and unequal. When good jobs are scarce, those from more affluent backgrounds can draw on reserves of economic, social and cultural capital to gain advantages over their peers (Crompton, 2010).

Mijs (2019) suggests that it is a paradox of inequality that the more rigid and unequal a society is, the more likely it is that the dominant culture in that society will promote the idea that individual success is due to individual merit rather than inherited privilege, even when there is overwhelming evidence that, for the most part, wealth and privilege are passed down from one generation to the next. The flip side of these beliefs is the belief that the poor must therefore be lazy and inadequate. Thus the belief that we live in a meritocracy can also fuel prejudiced and punitive attitudes towards the disadvantaged (Sandel, 2020). In recent years, rising levels of inequality have been accompanied by a growth in these negative attitudes towards the poor. We look at poverty and poverty stigma next.

REFLECTION POINT

We have seen that it is very difficult to move out of the class into which you were born. How helpful do you think Bourdieu's ideas of social and cultural capital are in explaining this low level of social mobility? Can you think of examples from your own experience?

Poverty

According to the Joseph Rowntree Foundation (JRF), poverty means not being able to meet minimum needs (JRF, 2020). There are two definitions of poverty. First, destitution or **absolute poverty**, refers to the level of poverty experienced by people who do not have the basic necessities required to survive. These are people who lack adequate food, clothing, heating and shelter, such as the rough sleepers living on our city streets. Second, we talk about **relative poverty**. This refers to the situation faced by people who have much less in relative terms than other members of their society. We define these people as poor when their poverty shuts them out of participation in society, that is, when they cannot afford to live what is generally accepted as a 'normal' life. For example, in the UK, being poor may mean not being able to afford decent housing, a healthy diet, access to the internet, or the ability to give Christmas presents. During the pandemic, relative poverty put the disadvantaged at greater risk. For example, overcrowded housing and precarious employment made it difficult to avoid infection (Marmot & Allen, 2020). Relative poverty very often means not being able to afford to live in adequate housing or afford adequate heating. The case study of Ben (below) gives a good example of the negative psychological and health effects of being shut out of normal life by poverty.

Case Example: Child Poverty

> *Eight-year-old Ben lives with his mother and two brothers in an overcrowded ground floor flat. Shortly after the family moved in, a severe damp and mould problem developed. An environmental health inspector has declared the property unfit for human habitation on two separate occasions. 'It's the smell that's almost the worst thing. It's so bad when you come into the flat' describes Ben's mother, Sandra. The damp and mould is having a severe impact on the children's health, which is affecting*

their education because they are missing school so often due to illness… The children's mental health is also being affected. Ben is being teased at school because his clothes smell of damp, which is affecting his self-confidence. 'It's not right…to be told that you smell. Kids are so cruel. [Ben] was teased for it. He's seeing the child psychologist now because he has low self-esteem'. The condition of the house makes it difficult for him to have friends round to play, which is impacting on his social development. 'When my friend comes round he says [my home] stinks and when I go to school this boy says my clothes stink … but Mummy washes them. (Ben aged eight)

(HARKER, 2006, p. 24)

This example is not untypical. Sadly, these problems are all too common, as figures show:

- 14 million people were living in poverty in 2020. This was made up of 8 million working-age adults, 4 million children and 2 million pensioners (JRF, 2020).
- A further 1.5 million people were considered to be destitute (Fitzpatrick et al., 2020).
- The majority (56%) of people in poverty are part of a working family (JRF, 2020).

In-work poverty is a growing problem that is being driven by the rise in precarious working described earlier. Many people in precarious work also move in and out of employment, and this group forms a significant proportion of people on benefits. While family poverty is increasing, so too is pensioner poverty (JRF, 2020). The disabled are at even greater risk of poverty than the able bodied, with a third of people with disabilities living in poverty (JRF, 2020).

Poverty has considerably increased in the last 10 years, and this has been exacerbated by the cuts in public services and welfare benefits brought in following the banking crisis of 2007–2008. Apart from cuts in benefits, we have seen a decline in community facilities such as libraries and youth centres. The ethos of austerity led, in the first two decades of the 21st century, to growing attempts to blame and shame the poor for their plight. This was expressed through the demonization of the poor in newspapers, news documentaries and reality shows, and this has led to increased class prejudice among the general public, with the poor described in some media as lazy, inadequate and living on 'hand-outs' (Valentine & Harris, 2013). We will talk a little more about the stigma of poverty in the next section.

POVERTY STIGMA

STIGMA

The concept of stigma describes treating someone negatively because of a perceived 'attribute' that is seen as 'discrediting,' such as poverty, obesity or disability. A stigmatised person (or group) is seen as having a 'tainted' and 'discredited' identity and is no longer treated as a 'whole' or 'usual' person (Goffman, 2009). Stigma can lead to ostracism, abuse, status loss and discrimination. Stigma is discussed in depth in Chapter 7.

As we saw in the previous section, people who are poor frequently have to do without things others consider necessities, such as decent housing or adequate heating. They can also face the chronic stress associated with insecure work and the constant struggle to make ends meet. They may be forced to live in the least desirable neighbourhoods in our towns and cities, where facilities are poor. However, instead of receiving sympathy for their difficult living conditions, there is increasing evidence that those living in poverty face stigma and are blamed for their predicament.

We can also see poverty stigma as a form of **'symbolic violence'** as described by Bourdieu in that denigrating and blaming the poor is used to justify growing inequality and declining welfare support (Thomas et al., 2020). This stigmatising discourse frequently distorts reality. For example, despite the fact that a majority of those who are poor are at work, the poor are represented in the media as workless scroungers (Valentine & Harris, 2014). This leads to hostility and prejudice. Alongside this discourse, public policies towards the poor, such as benefits and housing regulations, have become increasingly punitive (Wacquant, 2009). Snoussi and Mompelat (2019) reported that poor Londoners experienced prejudice and felt voiceless and dehumanised in their contact with statutory services including some health services.

Jones (2020) captured this contempt for the working-class poor in his book *Chavs: The Demonisation of the Working Class*. He suggests that demonising people at the bottom of society has long been seen as a convenient way to justify inequality. Taylor-Gooby (2013) has suggested that the public's declining sympathy for the poor can be directly related to media discourse but also reflects their lack of knowledge about the true extent of inequality.

There has been evidence of growing poverty stigma from a number of studies (Mooney, 2011). Several studies have shown that people living in social housing can face considerable prejudice that can affect many areas of their lives, including their ability to obtain work. We saw evidence of these prejudices in the aftermath of the Grenfell Tower fire (Shildrick, 2018). What matters to us as health workers is that these attitudes are not carried over into the treatment of patients from poorer backgrounds. However, there is evidence that many health professionals have little understanding of the life situations of their poorer patients and some clinicians can be prejudiced and judgmental (Tang, 2015; Wittenauer et al., 2015). We look at the impact of inequality on health next.

REFLECTION POINT

Go back to the case example of Ben. How do you think the stigma of poverty has affected his life? What was being done to help him? Was this likely to be effective? What else do you think could be done to combat the impact of poverty stigma on his life? How do you think that poverty stigma should be tackled in healthcare settings?

What Do We Know About the Impact of Social Inequalities on Health?

WORSENING INEQUALITIES

There has long been an understanding that wealth and poverty affect health. The first government study on health inequalities in the UK was produced in 1980 by Sir Douglas Black (DHSS, 1980). This was the first major piece of research to show conclusively that class affects your chances of living a long and healthy life. The report demonstrated that people in the poorest social classes suffered worse health at all stages of life. It also demonstrated a **'social gradient'** in that people in the middle class had worse health than the people at the top of the class hierarchy and better health than people nearer the bottom of the class hierarchy. The Black report suggested that inequality caused preventable deaths and that tackling health inequalities could save at least 17,000 lives every year. More recently the Marmot Review (Marmot et al., 2010) not only confirmed the findings of these earlier reports but also suggested that inequalities had worsened. In 2020, an updated review by Marmot showed a further 'worrying deterioration' in health inequalities even before the COVID-19 pandemic (Marmot et al., 2020). These inequalities adversely affected mortality rates during the pandemic, with the most deprived areas of the country experiencing the highest death rates from COVID-19 (Marmot & Allen, 2020).

INEQUALITIES IN LIFE EXPECTANCY

In 2010, the people of Glasgow had an average life expectancy of 74.3 years compared to 88.7 years for those living in the Royal Borough of Kensington and Chelsea (Dorling, 2013). This figure reflected regional inequalities which were linked to social class differences in different parts of Britain. In addition, there were also marked inequalities within localities linked to class differences. The difference in life expectancy for men between the richest and poorest areas within each local borough was more than 9 years for over 50% of the boroughs in England. Westminster had a 17-year within-area gap between the life expectancy of the richest and poorest residents. This was the highest in England, reflecting the stark differences between rich and poor in many parts of London (Marmot & Bell, 2012). Marmot also showed that people from the poorest parts of Britain were twice as likely to die before retirement when compared to those living in the most affluent neighbourhoods (Marmot et al., 2010).

As well as looking at class differences by comparing rich and poor areas of the country, we also can look directly at class differences in mortality by looking at an individual's occupation using measures like NS-SEC. Here, we see marked inequalities in life expectancy when comparing those in unskilled jobs with those in professional and managerial occupations. This mirrors the area data discussed above (Ingleby et al., 2021).

According to Marmot, health inequalities are 'not confined to poor health for the poor and good health for everyone else' (Marmot et al., 2020, p. 7). Everyone below the most affluent in society has a worse chance of living to an advanced age when compared to those at the top. However, the most deprived in society suffer the greatest threat of premature death (Marmot et al., 2020).

INEQUALITIES IN LONG-TERM ILLNESS AND DISABILITY

We have shown that class differences can affect life expectancy. There is a similar gradient in relation to your chances of suffering from a long-term, disabling illness before you reach retirement age. The chance of living in good health into old age is an important measure of the quality of people's lives and we call this **healthy life expectancy**.

- On average, in 2017, men spent 16.2 years (20.2%) of their lives in poor health. The figure for women was 19.4 years (23.3%).
- Women in the most deprived one-tenth of the population spent 34% of their lives in ill health. The figure for women in the most affluent one-tenth of the population was only 18%. The figures for men were 30% and 15% (Marmot et al., 2020, p. 23).

Deprivation greatly extends the number of years that you are likely to have to live in poor health. This means many people in the less affluent sections of the population start experiencing poor health long before retirement, while their more wealthy fellow citizens may be able to plan for a healthy retirement full of new leisure opportunities. Apart from its impact on people's quality of life, the number of years that people spend in poor health has an important impact on the demand for healthcare.

INFANT AND CHILD MORTALITY AND ILLNESS

Between March 2022 and March 2023, there were 3743 child deaths in England, and one-fifth of these were avoidable (National Child Mortality Database, 2023). Infant and child mortality has been increasing since 2014, and this increase has been linked to increases in child poverty. Babies born into families in the poorest one-tenth of the population have almost double the chance of dying in childhood when compared to babies from more wealthy families. The under-5 mortality rate in the UK was the second highest in Western Europe in 2019 (Taylor Robinson et al., 2019).

Children in the most deprived sections of the population are also more likely to face a serious or disabling illness during childhood. Factors adversely affecting children's ability to thrive during childhood include poverty, unemployment, homelessness, poor housing and parents' own poor physical and mental health (Marmot et al., 2020). Mental health problems also often start in childhood, with children from poorer backgrounds feeling less optimistic and having a greater sense of failure than their more affluent classmates. This may result from a feeling that they cannot live up to societal expectations and 'fit in' in terms of dress, appearance and school attainment (Mowat, 2019). They may also experience poverty stigma. We saw this in an earlier section in the case of Ben.

INEQUALITIES IN MENTAL HEALTH AND WELLBEING

People in poorer social classes are exposed to more stressors in their daily lives, whether this is the struggle to make ends meet, poor working conditions, poor housing or living in deprived neighbourhoods with poor services and high levels of crime. We talked earlier about how poverty involves having less than is needed to live a 'normal' life in a particular society. People in poverty can feel shut out of normal society, as they cannot afford to participate in activities that others take for granted, such as visiting a cinema or taking their children to a play centre. We call this experience of being shut out of normal society '**social exclusion**', and it has negative effects on both physical and mental wellbeing.

Thus social deprivation is associated with a higher prevalence of psychosis, depression, anxiety, substance misuse and suicide (Murali & Oyebode, 2004).

- Between 2017 and 2020, the proportion of adults experiencing anxiety or depression in the poorest one-fifth of the UK population was 26%. The figure for the next poorest one-fifth of the population was 22%, showing a **social gradient** in poor mental health.
- The level of anxiety and depression for the most affluent one-fifth of the population was only 13% (half that of the poorest one-fifth) (JRF, 2021).

We will talk in more detail about the psychosocial impacts of inequality in the next section when we discuss the explanations for socioeconomic inequalities in health.

Explaining Inequalities in Health

The reasons for health inequalities have been hotly debated for over four decades since the publication of the 'Black Report' (DHSS, 1980). Clearly, it is important that we understand the causes of a problem such as health inequality if we are going to tackle it effectively. It is likely that there are multiple causes of health inequalities but that some are more significant than others.

The Black Report considered four different explanations which people had put forward to explain the differences in health and life expectancy between different socio economic (class) groups (DHSS, 1980). The first suggestion made by some authors was that this finding was an '**artefact**'; in other words, just an error in the statistics caused by the difficulties of measuring abstract concepts such as health and social class. However, researchers have now measured health inequalities in many different ways. Studies have compared people in different occupations, and they have also compared rich and poor neighbourhoods, people living in different types of housing and people with different amounts of wealth and income. The authors of the Black Report rejected the artefact explanation, and the wealth of evidence that has been produced since 1980 leaves little reasonable doubt that the existence of health inequalities is real and not just a trick of the statistics (Marmot et al., 2010).

The second explanation that was considered in the Black Report was '**social selection**'. This theory suggests that we reverse the causal order and see health as influencing class position rather than assuming that class position affects health. This is a sociological version of Darwin's idea of the 'survival of the fittest'. This theory suggests that unhealthy people move down into the poorer social classes because they are unhealthy and therefore unproductive workers, while the healthiest members of society climb to the top. The first objection that we might make to this explanation is that it cannot be applied to inequalities in health during childhood. Second, we noted above that social mobility in the UK is very low and that most people do similar jobs to those of their parents. Studies have consistently failed to support the social selection theory. For example, the Whitehall studies, which are large-scale, longitudinal studies of civil servants, showed that health had no impact on changes in employment grade (Chandola et al., 2003).

There were just two remaining explanations which the Black Report authors thought were useful in explaining health inequalities. The first explanation was that people's health was influenced by their **material circumstances.** The second of these was the idea that people in different social classes have different **lifestyles and behaviours** which affect their health. These have been the most influential explanations for health inequalities and we will consider them in detail next. Then, we will look at a more recent explanation linking health inequalities to social stress.

MATERIAL CIRCUMSTANCES

We know that there is a social gradient in relation to access to wealth and all the health advantages that go with it. Thus, people in the poorer sections of society experience multiple sources of disadvantage and many of these are damaging to their health.

For example, we know that people in the poorer social classes are more likely to suffer from food insecurity (Marmot et al., 2010). According to Marmot (2020), between 8% and 10% of the UK population face difficulties affording enough to eat. The enormous growth in food banks in the UK is testament to the sharp rise in food insecurity since the previous report by Marmot in 2010 (Marmot et al., 2020). Apart from the risk of malnutrition, food insecurity can make it impossible to make healthy food choices.

We also know that the poorer members of our society suffer from fuel poverty and are unable to heat their homes sufficiently to stay healthy. Cold homes can contribute to excess winter mortality, particularly among the elderly. It can also contribute to respiratory illnesses, particularly when associated with damp housing. Lack of warm housing has been shown to adversely affect the mental health of all age groups (Marmot et al., 2020). Fuel poverty can also be closely associated with the health-damaging effects of poor housing. We saw these in the case study of Ben earlier. Poor housing can damage physical and mental health by exposing its inhabitants to hazards such as dampness, cold, mould, noise, overcrowding and fire risks (Marmot et al., 2020).

Poorer people can also find themselves living in what Marmot calls **'ignored places'**. These are places subject to what (Wacquant et al., 2016) call **'territorial stigmatisation'** where people can become 'urban outcasts'. Poorer areas often have poorer infrastructure, such as transport and shops, and greater exposure to environmental hazards such as heavy traffic and poor air quality. They are less likely to have access to green spaces and leisure facilities. Marmot suggests that these ignored places are more likely to have seen cuts in public services such as schools, health services, libraries and sports facilities. (see also Chapter 4). According to Marmot, these 'ignored areas' are most likely to be found in the post-industrial north and coastal towns, as we noted in our earlier discussion of geographical inequality (Marmot et al., 2020). Poorer areas often also have worse health services. The public health doctor Julian Tudor Hart described this inequity as the **'inverse care law'** (Hart, 1971). He suggested that the provision of health services displayed an inverse relationship with the need for those services. For example, both inner-city areas and rural areas often have high levels of deprivation but fewer services than more affluent suburbs and small towns.

When we talk about material deprivation, we are not just talking about people's living conditions but also their working conditions. Both poor-quality work and unemployment can cause ill health. There are significant health hazards involved in many occupations, such as workplace accidents and poor air quality, but the most widely reported adverse consequences of work involve chronic stress due to long hours, heavy workloads, poor working relationships and low pay. Work stress accounts for increasing amounts of mental and physical illness. In addition, we know that unemployment adversely affects health (Marmot et al., 2020).

BEHAVIOUR LIFESTYLE AND CULTURE

When we talk about unhealthy lifestyles, we are talking about things like poor diet, consumption of tobacco and alcohol, and lack of exercise. We all know that these things are bad for us, but to what extent is it true that people who are less well-off are more likely to engage in these unhealthy behaviours? What studies of health and lifestyles have shown is that people across all classes in society understand the messages about healthy and unhealthy lifestyles, such as 'exercise more' and 'eat 5 a day', so it is not lack of education that stops people from quitting unhealthy behaviours. For example, a key study on health and lifestyles showed that people throughout society were aware of healthy messages and that a whole variety of factors influenced healthy and unhealthy choices (Blaxter, 2003).

Blaxter (2003) also showed that people in poorer circumstances got fewer health benefits from making healthy choices. This was because the health-damaging effects of adverse life circumstances such as poor housing and poverty tended to overshadow any improvements in lifestyle that they were able to make. Blaxter thus showed that the health gains from taking up healthy behaviours such as exercise were far greater for the better-off. Thus, making healthy choices is harder for people in adverse circumstances due both to a lack of resources and chronic stress and the payoff is often smaller.

Marmot (2010) has suggested that differences in lifestyle account for only about one-third of the differences in morbidity and mortality between the social classes. A number of studies have also confirmed that a lack of resources makes it more difficult to make healthy choices. For example, a healthy diet is expensive. Marmot (2020) reported that people in the poorest one-tenth of society would have to spend three-quarters of their disposable income on food to meet government healthy eating guidelines, whereas the wealthiest one-tenth would only have to spend 6%.

PSYCHOSOCIAL FACTORS

We noted at the start of this chapter that the classical sociologist Max Weber described social class as having three facets: (1) how much money you have, (2) how much status and respect you receive and (3) how much power and control over your life you have.. Recently, researchers have started to think more about these latter two aspects of class, namely respect and control, and examine their impact on health. Marmot's large-scale longitudinal study of Whitehall civil servants found that a **social gradient** in health existed throughout all the grades of civil servants. None of these people were poor, but even the lower grades of the civil service had a shorter life expectancy than the higher grades. Marmot concluded that this social gradient was due to differences in working conditions and, in particular, suggested that a lack of social support and a low level of control at work were linked to worse health (Marmot, 2004). Siegrist and Marmot (2004) elaborated this argument further by suggesting that high demands at work and low control (which is called '**job strain**') and the demoralisation of what they called '**effort-reward imbalance**' (i.e. having to work hard for comparatively low rewards) were detrimental to both mental and physical health.

Wilkinson and Pickett (2009) have argued that wealthy societies with high levels of inequality, such as the UK, experience higher levels of relative deprivation. This leads to a decline in social cohesion and trust across the whole of society. Pickett and Wilkinson suggest that the populations of highly unequally wealthy countries, as a result, have a worse life expectancy than more equal societies with the same level of wealth. They suggest that this is partly because poorer people in highly unequal societies, such as the UK, experience more psychosocial stress. This is due to a lack of social support, not having the power and resources to control their material circumstances and being stigmatised and made to feel inferior in many social situations. These situations include interactions with teachers, health professionals, the police, benefits agencies, housing agencies and employers (Pickett & Wilkinson, 2010). There are clear links here with Bourdieu's concept of 'symbolic violence'.

We noted earlier in the chapter that people from poorer backgrounds can experience stigma, victim blaming, social exclusion and 'symbolic violence'. The case study of Ben showed how his poverty and poor housing led to experiences of stigma, which were already affecting his mental health at a young age. These negative experiences can then accumulate across the life course, with poorer people experiencing stigma at school, at work and in contact with a range of service providers, including healthcare workers. The life course approach to health inequalities has suggested that a combination of material circumstances, lifestyle factors and psychosocial stresses combine across a lifetime to produce ill health (Bartley, 2016).

REFLECTION POINT

Review the explanations of the health inequalities outlined above. How helpful do you think the final explanation is? List examples of psychosocial stressors that you think could be health damaging. Can you find evidence to support your ideas?

TACKLING HEALTH INEQUALITIES

The solutions that governments have pursued to tackle health inequalities have only been partially influenced by evidence. Political factors have frequently played a pivotal role in decisions about which policies will be implemented (Calnan, 2020). In recent years, despite much rhetoric and many well-meaning schemes to tackle health inequalities, the problem has been getting worse, and this has now been accelerated by the COVID-19 pandemic (Dorling, 2020).

Tackling health inequalities requires tackling unequal exposure to health risks throughout society, for example in workplaces, housing and local neighbourhoods. It means comprehensively addressing the social determinants of health outlined in Chapter 1. However, governments frequently place most of their focus on individual lifestyles (Calnan, 2020). As a consequence, they also place much of the responsibility for tackling health inequalities on health and social care professionals. As we noted in Chapter 1, we need more 'upstream' thinking, and this is, to some extent, a 'downstream' solution. The Marmot (2010) review suggested that to tackle health inequalities, every child needs to be given a good start in life, people need to be given more control over their lives, better jobs need to be created to give everyone a healthy standard of living, communities need better support and preventive health needs to be strengthened.

This chapter has presented evidence to show that much of the health disadvantage suffered by poorer people is due to material conditions that are very difficult for individuals to control. Lifestyles are hard to change for all of us, but they are an extreme challenge when you are experiencing adverse social circumstances that you do not have the power to change. As health professionals, we also need to be aware that there are psychosocial stresses associated with feeling disrespected and powerless that can affect a person's health. These are stresses that health professionals can exacerbate through insensitive behaviour and patronising or stigmatising attitudes.

Summary of Key Points

- Levels of social class inequality in the UK are high compared to many other developed countries and are increasing.
- This inequality leads to avoidable morbidity and mortality.
- Material deprivation has the greatest impact on inequalities in health.
- While behaviour and lifestyle are also important causes of health inequalities, they are less important than material deprivation.
- The psychosocial stresses associated with being unable to control your life circumstances and feeling inferior and stigmatised also exert a toll on people's physical and mental health.
- Adverse material circumstances, lifestyle and psychosocial stresses are closely interwoven in their effects on health and need to be tackled together.

Further Reading

Jones, O. (2020). *Chavs: The demonization of the working class*. Verso.

Dorling, D. (2013). *Unequal health: The scandal of our times*. Policy Press.

Marmot, M., & Bell, R. (2012). Fair society. *healthy lives. Public Health, 126*, 4–12.

Snoussi, D., & Mompelat, L. (2019). *We are ghosts': Race, class and institutional prejudice*. Runnymede Trust.

References

Ahmed, N., Marriott, A., Dabi, N., Lowthers, M., Lawson, M., & Mugehera, L. (2022). *Inequality kills: The unparalleled action needed to combat unprecedented inequality in the wake of COVID-19*. Oxfam.

Bartley, M. (2016). *Health inequality: An introduction to concepts, theories and methods*. John Wiley & Sons.

Blaxter, M. (2003). *Health and lifestyles*. Routledge.

Bourdieu, P. (1984). *Distinction: A social critique of the judgement of taste*. Harvard University Press.

Calnan, M. (2020). *Health policy, power and politics: Sociological insights*. Emerald Publishing Limited.

Causa, O., & Johansson, A. (2009). *Intergenerational social mobility: Working paper no 707*. Organisation for Economic Cooperation and Development. Retrieved November 28, 2023, from. https://www.oecd-ili-brary.org/economics/intergenerational-social-mobility_223106258208.

Chandola, T., Bartley, M., Sacker, A., Jenkinson, C., & Marmot, M. (2003). Health selection in the Whitehall II study. *UK. Social Science & Medicine, 56*(10), 2059–2072.

Christensen, M. B., Hallum, C., Maitland, A., Parrinello, Q., & Putaturo, C. (2023). *Survival of the richest: How we must tax the super-rich now to fight inequality*. Oxfam.

Crompton, R. (2010). Class and employment. Work. *Employment and Society, 24*(1), 9–26.

Delestre, I., Kopczuk, W., Miller, H., Smith, K. (2022), 'Top income inequality and tax policy', IFS deaton review of inequalities. https://ifs.org.uk/inequality/top-income-inequality-and-tax-policy.

Department of Health and Social Security. (1980). *Inequalities in health: Report of a research working group*. Department of Health and Social Security.

Dorling, D. (2013). *Unequal health: The scandal of our times*. Policy Press.

Dorling, D. (2018). *Peak Inequality*. Policy Press.

Dorling, D. (2019). *Inequality and the 1%*. Verso.

Dorling, D. (2020). *COVID-19: The rise in destitution and inequality in the UK* (pp. 14–17). Public Sector Focus. July/August. https://www.dannydorling.org/?p=7960.

Equality Trust. (2021). Pay ratios. Retrieved December 13, 2023, from https://www.equalitytrust.org.uk/taxonomy/term/136.

Fitzpatrick, S., Bramley, G., Blenkinsopp, J., Wood, J., Sosenko, F., Littlewood, M., Johnsen, S., Watts, B., Treanor, M., & McIntyre, J. (2020). *Destitution in the UK 2020*. Joseph Rowntree Foundation.

Gerth, H. H., & Mills, C. W. (2014). *From Max Weber: Essays in sociology*. Routledge.

Giddens, A., & Sutton, P. W. (2021). *Sociology*. John Wiley & Sons.

Goffman, E. (2009). *Stigma: Notes on the management of spoiled identity*. Simon and Schuster.

Harker, L. (2006). Delivering on child poverty: What would it take? A report for the department for work and pensions Vol. 6951. The Stationery Office.

Hart, J. T. (1971). The inverse care law. *The Lancet, 297*(7696), 405–412.

Heath, S. (2007). Widening the gap: Pre-university gap years and the 'economy of experience. *British Journal of Sociology of Education, 28*(1), 89–103.

Hecht, K., McArthur, D., Savage, M., & Friedman, S. (2020). *Elites in the UK: Pulling away? Social mobility, geographic mobility and elite occupations*. The Sutton Trust.

High Pay Centre. (2023). FTSE 100 CEOs' earnings for 2023 will surpass the median UK worker's full time annual salary today, just prior to 14:00 on Thursday 5 January. Retrieved December 13, 2023, from https://highpaycentre.org/high-pay-hour-how-quickly-ceos-earn-the-uk-median-wage/.

Hills, J., Brewer, M., Jenkins, S., Lister, R., Lupton, R., Machin, S., Mills, C., Modood, T., Rees, T., & Riddell, S. (2010). *An anatomy of economic inequality in the UK: Report of the national equality panel*. Government Equalities Office.

Hudson, R. (2013). Thatcherism and its geographical legacies: The new map of socio-spatial inequality in the Divided Kingdom. *The Geographical Journal, 179*(4), 377–381.

Ingleby, F. C., Woods, L. M., Atherton, I. M., Baker, M., Elliss-Brookes, L., & Belot, A. (2021). Describing socio-economic variation in life expectancy according to an individual's education, occupation and wage in England and Wales: An analysis of the ONS longitudinal study. *SSM-Population Health, 14*, 100815.

Jones, O. (2020). *Chavs: The demonization of the working class.* Verso.

Joseph Rowntree Foundation. (2020). UK poverty 2019/20. www.jrf.org.uk.

Joseph Rowntree Foundation. (2021). UK poverty statistics. Retrieved May 23, 2021, from https://www.jrf.org.uk/data/adults-experiencing-anxiety-or-depression-income-group.

Lansley, S., & Mack, J. (2015). *Breadline Britain: The rise of mass poverty.* Simon and Schuster.

Marmot, M. G. (2004). *Status syndrome: How your social standing directly affects your health and life expectancy.* Bloomsbury Publishing.

Marmot, M., Allen, J., Goldblatt, P., Boyce, T., McNeish, D., Grady, M., & Geddes, I. (2010). *The marmot review: Fair society, healthy lives.* University College London.

Marmot, M., Allen, J., Boyce, T., Goldblatt, E., & Morrison, J. (2020). *Health equity in England: The marmot review 10 years on.* Institute of Health Equity.

Marmot, M., & Allen, J. (2020). COVID-19: Exposing and amplifying inequalities. *Journal of Epidemiology & Community Health, 74,* 681–682.

Marmot, M., & Bell, R. (2012). Fair society. *healthy lives. Public Health, 126,* 4–12.

Marx, K. (2016). Economic and philosophic manuscripts of 1844. In Longhofer, W., & Winchester, D. (Eds.), *Social theory re-wired* (pp. 142–147). Routledge.

Mijs, J. J. (2019). The paradox of inequality: Income inequality and belief in meritocracy go hand in hand. *Socio-Economic Review, 19*(1), 7–35.

Mooney, G. (2011). *Stigmatising poverty? The 'Broken Society' and reflections on anti-welfarism in the UK today.* Oxfam.

Mowat, J. G. (2019). Exploring the impact of social inequality and poverty on the mental health and wellbeing and attainment of children and young people in Scotland. *Improving Schools, 22*(3), 204–223.

Muntaner, C. (2018). Digital platforms, gig economy, precarious employment, and the invisible hand of social class. *International Journal of Health Services, 48*(4), 597–600.

Murali, V., & Oyebode, F. (2004). Poverty, social inequality and mental health. *Advances in Psychiatric Treatment, 10*(3), 216–224.

National Child Mortality Database. (2023). Child death review data release: Year ending 31 March 2023. Retrieved December 2, 2023, from https://www.ncmd.info/publications/child-death-data-2023/.

Office for National Statistics (ONS). (2010). The national statistics socio-economic classification (NS-SEC). Retrieved December 12, 2023, from https://www.ons.gov.uk/methodology/classificationsandstandards/otherclassifications/thenationalstatisticssocioeconomicclassificationnssecrebasedonsoc2010.

ONS. (2013). 2011 Census: Key statistics and quick statistics for local authorities in the United Kingdom. Retrieved December 12, 2023, from https://www.ons.gov.uk/employmentandlabourmarket/peopleinwork/employmentandemployeetypes/bulletins/keystatisticsandquickstatisticsforlocalauthorities-intheunitedkingdom/2013-12-04.

ONS. (2019). Total wealth in Great Britain: April 2016 to March 2018. Retrieved December 12, 2023, from https://www.ons.gov.uk/peoplepopulationandcommunity/personalandhouseholdfinances/incomeandwealth/bulletins/totalwealthingreatbritain/latest.

Organisation for Economic Cooperation and Development (OECD). (2016). *Factbook 2015–2016 economic, environmental and social statistics.* OECD.

Pickett, K., & Wilkinson, R. (2010). *The spirit level.* Penguin Books.

Piketty, T. (2014). *Capital in the twenty-first century.* Harvard University Press.

Reay, D. (2013). Social mobility, a panacea for austere times: Tales of emperors, frogs, and tadpoles. *British Journal of Sociology of Education, 34*(5–6), 660–677.

Rowlingson, K., & McKay, S. (2013). *What Do the Public Think about the Wealth Gap?* University of Birmingham.

Sandel, M. J. (2020). *The tyranny of merit: What's become of the common good?* Macmillan.

Savage, M. (2015). *Social class in the 21st century.* Penguin.

Silva, E., & Warde, A. (2010). *Cultural analysis and Bourdieu's legacy: Settling accounts and developing alternatives.* Routledge.

Shildrick, T., & MacDonald, R. (2013). Poverty talk: How people experiencing poverty deny their poverty and why they blame 'the poor. *The Sociological Review, 61*(2), 285–303.

Shucksmith, J., Carlebach, S., Riva, M., Curtis, S., Hunter, D., Blackman, T., & Hudson, R. (2010). *Health inequalities in ex-coalfield/industrial communities.* Local Government Association.

Siegrist, J., & Marmot, M. (2004). Health inequalities and the psychosocial environment—two scientific challenges. *Social Science & Medicine, 58*(8), 1463–1473.

Snoussi, D., & Mompelat, L. (2019). *We are ghosts': Race, class and institutional prejudice*. Runnymede Trust.

Standing, G. (2014). The precariat—The new dangerous class. *Amalgam, 6*(6–7), 115–119.

Sutton Trust and Social Mobility Commission. (2019). Elitist Britain 2019. The educational backgrounds of Britain's leading people. Retrieved December 2, 2023, from https://www.suttontrust.com/our-research/elitist-britain-2019/.

Tang, Y., Browne., A. J., Mussell, B., Smye, V. L., & Rodney, P. (2015). 'Underclassism'and access to healthcare in urban centres. *Sociology of Health & Illness, 37*(5), 698–714.

Taylor-Gooby, P. (2013). Why do people stigmatise the poor at a time of rapidly increasing inequality, and what can be done about it? *The Political Quarterly, 84*(1), 31–42.

Taylor-Robinson, D., Lai, E. T., Wickham, S., Rose, T., Norman, P., Bambra, C., & Barr, B. (2019)Assessing the impact of rising child poverty on the unprecedented rise in infant mortality in England, 2000–2017: Time trend analysis9. BMJ Open, e029424.

Thomas, F., Wyatt, K., & Hansford, L. (2020). The violence of narrative: Embodying responsibility for poverty-related stress *Sociology of Health & Illness, 42*(5), 1123–1138.

Toft, M., & Friedman, S. (2020). Family wealth and the class ceiling: The propulsive power of the bank of Mum and Dad. *Sociology, 55*(1), 1–20.

Valentine, G., & Harris, C. (2014). Strivers vs. skivers: Class prejudice and the demonisation of dependency in everyday life. *Geoforum, 53*, 84–92.

Wacquant, L. (2009). *Punishing the poor: The neoliberal government of social insecurity*. Duke University Press.

Wacquant, L. (2016). Revisiting territories of relegation: Class, ethnicity and state in the making of advanced marginality. *Urban Studies, 53*(6), 1077–1088.

Wilkinson, R. G., & Pickett, K. E. (2009). Income inequality and social dysfunction. *Annual Review of Sociology, 35*, 493–511.

Wittenauer, J., Ludwick, R., Baughman, K., & Fishbein, R. (2015). Surveying the hidden attitudes of hospital nurses' towards poverty. *Journal of Clinical Nursing, 24*(15–16), 2184–2191.

World Inequality Lab. (2018). World inequality report. Retrieved December 12, 2023, from https://wir2018.wid.world/.

Gender Inequalities in Health

This chapter will examine gender inequalities and how they impact on health. It will look, firstly, at what we mean by the term *gender* and how this differs from biological sex. It will then consider how gender is socially constructed. It will examine inequalities based on gender identity within society and consider the different forms of disadvantage that can result from these, focusing primarily on the position of women in society. It will examine gender differences in mortality and morbidity and the reasons for these. It will then consider men and women's experiences of healthcare and how these have been shaped historically by a view of male physiology as the norm and women's physiology as a deviation from this. The chapter will then look at how this has affected the treatment of illnesses predominantly suffered by women. Finally, it will consider inequalities in health in relation to sexual and gender minorities, such as gay, lesbian and transgender people.

Changing Conceptions of Gender

Traditionally, it was believed that there were clear-cut differences between men and women and that these were based on biological differences. These biological differences were also presumed to account for differences in the behaviours of men and women and to determine the different roles that men and women should play in society. These beliefs arose in a society largely dominated and controlled by males in which public discourse was also controlled by men. This led to a fixed set of beliefs and values which defined the role of women as subordinate to men and confined most women to serving their family within a domestic environment. We will see this very clearly later in the chapter, when we look in more detail at how medical ideas about men and women's bodies developed over centuries.

In more recent history, the roles of men and women have been changing. Women over 30 with property first achieved the vote in the UK in 1918, but women only finally achieved the vote on equal terms with men in 1928. Women gradually began to achieve more social and political rights throughout the 20th century through legislation, such as the Equal Pay Act in 1970, Sex

Discrimination Act in 1975 and Equality Act in 2010. However, overturning the legacy of centuries of inequality has been slow. Before the 20th century, women were excluded from many areas of work and education; women were largely forbidden to attend university and to enter many occupations. It was considered that their biological sex rendered them mentally and physically inferior and thus incapable of an independent life outside the domestic sphere and the control of men.

For example, the first seven women to try to train to be doctors in the UK studied at the University of Edinburgh in 1869. They faced a campaign of hostility and abuse from male doctors and students culminating in the staging of a riot to prevent them from taking their exams during which the male students pelted them with mud and rubbish and released a live sheep into the examination hall. Remarkably, despite this level of harassment, the women still passed their exams. However, the University of Edinburgh refused to let the women graduate. The women brought a court case in 1873 to try to force the university to grant their degrees. The university won on the grounds that, as women, they were mentally and physically unfit to study at a university and thus should never have been allowed to join the University (Oxford Dictionary of Biography, 2004). One of these women, Sophia Jex Blake, became the first female doctor in the UK in 1877, but she had been forced to obtain her degree in Switzerland. Women's access to work and education gradually opened up throughout the 20th century as a result of the efforts of women like Sophia Jex Blake. However, progress was slow. For example, Cambridge University did not award degrees to women until 1948. As we shall see later, men still dominate many areas of public life and the upper ranks of many occupations.

The biological determinism which dominated thinking about men and women for centuries has declined in influence although it has not completely disappeared from academic and political discourse (Miller & Costello, 2001). However, there is now much more widespread agreement that the social roles that men and women play are not determined by their biological sex but socially constructed. Thus, they can vary over time and between different societies. Most contemporary women will live very different lives and perform very different social roles to their grandmothers and great grandmothers as many more women have joined the labour force over recent decades. We can therefore make a distinction between **biological sex** and **gender**. The term 'sex' is used to refer to biological differences between males and females. The term 'gender' is used to refer to the social identities of males and females and we can see these as **socially constructed**. Thus, gender refers to the different social roles, social identities and social behaviours associated with being male or female. As we discuss later in this section, gender is seen by many sociologists as a social construct and gender roles can vary and change over time.

Social constructionism is associated with 'micro' sociology (see Chapter 1) and refers to the ways in which social phenomena, social roles and identities are constructed through everyday social interactions. This shows how both our identities and our understanding of reality are shaped by culture throughout our lives. Thus, things we consider 'natural', such as gender identities, are actually socially defined and vary between time and place. Social constructionism challenges biological determinism's belief that it is our biology that determines our identity and destiny. Much of what we perceive as natural and self-evident reality is, in fact, shaped by shared social assumptions, and these assumptions can change over time as society changes. A key text outlining the theory of social constructionism was Thomas Berger and Peter Luckmann's book 'The Social Construction of Reality', published in 1967. We return to this concept in Chapters 5, 6 and 7.

People learn gender roles through gender socialisation which begins as soon as a baby is born and is often expressed through the different ways in which people talk to boy and girl babies, as well as the use of gender-specific toys and clothing. Children gradually learn the norms and expectations associated with their assigned gender through family, school, the wider community and various social agencies including the media. Gender-stereotyped products can also be big business and can be intensively marketed through gender-specific products for babies and children, such as toys, books, computer games and clothing. Gender stereotypes can be, on the one hand, pervasive and obtrusive, but on the other hand can also be very subtly conveyed. This means that even parents wanting to avoid gender stereotyping in the upbringing of their children can find it hard to escape. However, interactionist sociologists have pointed out that gender socialisation is not a deterministic process, and although the pressures to conform to gender stereotypes are powerful, they can be and are resisted to some degree (Giddens & Sutton, 2021). As gender roles and identities are socially constructed, we should expect them to change as society changes, although, at the same time, some gendered expectations and stereotypes do seem to be remarkably sticky and persistent. An interesting example of the subtleties of gender socialisation can be found in a study of absence due to sickness among primary school children. This study showed how expectations in relation to health behaviours differed for girls and boys (Prout, 1986). Prout found that boys tended to be regarded as 'wet' by teachers and parents if they complained of feeling ill, reinforcing the gender stereotype that boys should be brave and stoic. Girls, on the other hand, were frequently described as 'little actresses' whose claims of sickness were untrustworthy and emotionally manipulative. We will meet these attitudes again when we talk about gendered experiences in healthcare.

Whereas we used to regard gender identity as a simple dichotomy of male versus female, there is now growing recognition that gender is, in reality, a more fluid concept (Annandale & Hunt, 2000). It can be more helpful to think of gender identity as a continuum of what have traditionally been thought of as 'typically' male and female characteristics and behaviours. It has been increasingly recognised, for example, that some people can have a deeply felt sense of gender identity which is at odds with the gender identity assigned to them at birth on the basis of their biological sex. There has been growing recognition of this sense of unease about the gender one has been assigned at birth and it has been labelled 'gender dysphoria' or 'gender incongruence' (WHO, 2016). At present, management of 'gender incongruence' in this country is largely medicalised in the same way as many other areas of social behaviour (Johnson, 2019) (we discuss medicalisation in Chapter 6). We use the term 'transgender' to refer to people who have transitioned away from the gender identity that they were assigned at birth on the basis of their biological sex. The term 'non-binary' is also used by people who regard their gender identity as not fitting either male or female gender identities. The precise numbers of people identifying themselves as either transgender or 'non-binary' as a result of gender dysphoria is unknown, but this is a fast-growing social phenomenon which is indicative of wider changes in gender roles within society.

A very small number of people are intersex in that they are born with variations in sex characteristics which make their gender identity ambiguous. This includes conditions such as Klinefelter syndrome and congenital adrenal hyperplasia. While genital abnormalities at birth may be relatively common and are estimated to occur in 1 out of 300 births in the UK, abnormalities which result in gender ambiguity are thought to be much rarer, occurring in around 1 out of 5000 births (Government Equalities Office, 2019). There are also variations and some fluidity in sexual orientation, and in this book we will use the term *sexual and gender minorities* (SGM) to describe lesbian, gay, bisexual, transgender and other groups whose sexual orientation and gender expression differs from what has traditionally been seen as 'normal'.

Gender Inequalities in Society

This section will briefly outline evidence of the continuing presence of gender inequalities in society and the reasons for their continued existence. Firstly, it is clear that, despite many improvements in women's positions at work, women can still face inequality and disadvantages in the workplace. Despite it being over 50 years since the Equal Pay Act was first passed in the UK, there is still a gender pay gap in the UK with women, on average, earning 14.9% less than men in hourly earnings in 2022 (Statista, 2023). This persists despite girls' increasing success in education where they now often outperform boys. The gender pay gap between male and female graduates is 5% at aged 25, despite women being more likely to get a higher university degree. By the age of 30, this has widened to 25%, with the widest gender pay gap affecting women over 50 (Institute of Fiscal Studies, 2021). The 5% difference soon after graduation can be partly explained by men being more likely to choose subjects with a higher financial return which have traditionally been seen as 'masculine' subjects. However, this does not explain the widening gap over time. This may largely be explained by the fact that women's heavier responsibilities for unpaid care work in the home force them into part-time or full-time work that they can easily fit around these responsibilities.

Women are almost three times more likely to be in part-time work with 38% of women working part time compared to 13% of men (Buchanan et al., 2023). Women are more likely to be working in jobs paying the minimum wage and more likely to be living in persistent poverty (Buchanan et al., 2023). Lower pay and part-time work means women are less able to save for their retirement and have lower pensions. One fifth of retired women live in poverty and this rises to 27% of women living alone (Age UK, 2021). The distribution of income within families can also contribute to women's poverty. In some households, income is still controlled by men and the tax and benefit systems still often operate on the basis of a 'male breadwinner' model which can disadvantage women (Annesley & Bennett, 2011).

GENDER DISCRIMINATION AND 'EVERYDAY SEXISM'

Gender discrimination in the workplace remains an important reason for gender inequalities at work. Although the UK has now had three women prime ministers, men still dominate the upper echelons of most major organisations and businesses. For example, 96% of the chief executives of major UK corporations are men (Maddock Jones, 2022). Another important reason why women are disadvantaged in the workplace is that, as we have seen, they still carry more responsibility for unpaid work within the family, such as household management, childcare and care of older, sick and disabled family members. Caring has traditionally been seen as women's work' and still disproportionately falls on women's shoulders. This is an important reason for the higher proportion of part-time working amongst women, particularly middle-aged and older women. The working world has traditionally been, to a large extent, designed by men for men, and although the situation is improving, access to flexible working and childcare is still often inadequate, making it very difficult for many women to juggle their family responsibilities and a full-time job. State support for childcare has also been poor. This reflects the values of a society which devalues both paid and unpaid caring work leading both to be poorly esteemed and rewarded. It is largely women who pay the penalty for the fact that society does not value or reward caring work (Evans, 2017). For example, 80% of jobs in the social care sector are filled by women and jobs in social care are amongst the lowest-paid jobs in the UK economy (Skills for Care, 2010).

Another important driver of gender inequality is the continued existence of sexist attitudes towards women and the continued problems women face in dealing with everyday sexism, sexual harassment and, at worst, sexual violence. For example, on average, two women per week in the UK are killed by a male partner or ex-partner, while globally, six women per hour are killed by a partner or family member (World Economic Forum, 2020). Recent high-profile court cases have also uncovered the prolific sexual abuse of women by some powerful men in public life, such as Harvey Weinstein. This led to the creation of the 'Me Too' movement. This movement highlighted women's everyday experiences of sexual harassment and sexism and protested against these experiences (O'Neil et al., 2018). More than one in three women globally have experienced intimate partner or sexual violence, and this can often have negative consequences for women's physical, psychological and reproductive health (WHO, 2021a). According to the World Health Organization, violence against women is a major public health problem and health professionals have an important role to play in identifying and preventing it (WHO, 2021b).

Women still face everyday sexism and the risk of male violence in their day-to-day lives at school, work, in public places and in personal relationships (Bates, 2016). Older women also face abuse which combines sexism with ageism (Smith, 2023). Sexual harassment and everyday sexism in the workplace and educational settings can be a chronic stressor which both undermines women's health and negatively affects their performance in work and education (O'Neil et al., 2018). Below are some examples posted by women and girls on the 'The Everyday Sexism Project' website (2023):

Examples: Everyday Sexism

J: Despite handling the majority of correspondence and information gathering for my re-mortgage, our advisor put the account in my partner's name.

A: I injured my ankle and saw a doctor with my husband in the room… The doctor (who was a man) asked me if I worked and I replied that I was a teacher. The doctor wrote this up as, 'It was a pleasure to see Alice with her husband. She works in a play school.' I have loads of respect for anyone who works in a play school but I teach secondary maths.

V: I was admitted to hospital when I was 21 because I'd just been diagnosed with diabetes. I was very scared and upset and alone as I was at university. Whilst I was in a cubicle on my own in just a gown a youngish doctor came in and asked if I'd had a breast exam yet. I said no and he examined me and then went away without saying anything. I realised later that I'd been sexually assaulted https://everydaysexism.com/.

The feminist movement has focussed on the issue of sexism for many years but this was recently brought into sharper focus by the 'Me Too' movement. From a social determinants perspective it is important to address all the various sources of gender inequalities outlined above in order to improve the health status of women (O'Neil et al., 2018). We will look at the contribution of feminism next.

REFLECTION POINT

Think about your own experiences of being subject to or witnessing everyday sexism. What do you think the impact of these experiences might be on people's physical and mental health? How do you think that everyday sexism should be tackled in healthcare settings?

FEMINIST THEORY

Feminist theories began to come to prominence in the late 18th century in the work of Mary Wollstonecraft whose book 'A Vindication of the Rights of Women published in 1792 argued that females were not naturally inferior to males and should have the right to an education (Wollstonecraft, 2004). Feminist theories have sought to explain gender inequalities with reference to structural processes and social institutions, such as patriarchy, sexism and capitalism. Three traditions of feminist theory have been identified.

The first, often referred to as **'liberal feminism'**, is a reformist movement that tries to work within existing institutions to achieve gradual improvements to women's position in society by addressing issues, such as legal rights and equal opportunities. Its successes have included legislation, such as the Equal Pay Act 1970 (Bryson, 2016, 2021). Critics have argued that although liberal feminists have achieved some important gains and improved women's opportunities, they have not managed to address more ingrained issues, such as everyday sexism and the continued dominance of men in many areas of social and economic life. It has also been suggested by some authors that liberal feminism has mainly benefitted a small, elite group of better-off women (Carpenter, 2000).

Radical feminism focuses on what it describes as a system of patriarchy through which men systematically dominate and oppress women. It focuses attention on the ways in which patriarchal culture perpetuates women's subordination by, for example, promoting idealised forms of beauty and femininity which give primacy to pleasing and servicing men. Thus, radical feminists place more emphasis on the problem of sexism and male violence against women and see this as part of a wider culture of oppression (Bryson, 2016).

Socialist and Marxist feminists place more emphasis on the role of economic institutions and ideologies, such as neoliberalism (see Chapter 8) in creating gender inequalities. They see tackling gender inequality as part of a broader campaign for economic, social and political justice and place more emphasis on the structural causes of gender inequality. Evans, for example, argues that there are powerful commercial interests involved both in promoting gender stereotypes to sell products and also in ensuring that the care work mainly carried out by women remains unpaid and unrecognised (Evans, 2017).

INTERSECTIONALITY

The term 'intersectionality' was coined by Crenshaw in 1989 (Crenshaw, 2017) and it describes the ways in which different types of inequality and disadvantage can intersect. Thus, it tells us how systems of inequality, such as gender, race, class, sexual orientation, disability and age can interact with one another. Crenshaw initially coined the term to describe the particular experiences of Black women. These were different to those of White women in similar situations because they faced an additional layer of discrimination and disadvantage.

We saw earlier that the pay gap between men and women was 14.9%, but taking an intersectional perspective, we can also break this down by race. We then see that Black women earn on average 19.6% less than White men and so face additional disadvantage (Fawcett Society, 2019). Intersectionality sees an individual's social position as a particular spot in a matrix of intersecting systems of power. Take for example, two women experiencing poverty. One is an elderly working-class White woman, the other a middle aged, Black, disabled woman. Each might have some similar experiences of gender inequality, class inequality and poverty stigma but also some very different experiences, with the first woman likely to experience ageism and the second likely to experience both racism and disability discrimination. Taking a perspective that only considers one type of inequality can make us miss the ways that disadvantages can stack up in an individual's life. For example, Shifrer and Frederick (2019) have suggested that the disability rights movement has often ignored the additional discrimination faced by Black, disabled people. This (and other instances of intersecting disadvantage) can lead to people being left out of systems of support as well as being treated as 'exceptions' in antidiscrimination legislation.

Critics of the concept of intersectionality have pointed to its neglect of social class and have argued that this fragmented understanding of social identities may make it more difficult to understand and challenge institutionalised economic and political inequalities (Salem, 2018). However, within the health field it can be a useful adjunct to work on social determinants of health and can also be useful for understanding the different experiences of patients from different backgrounds (Gkiouleka et al., 2018). We will return to this concept in Chapter 4.

Gender and Health Inequality

GENDER DIFFERENCES IN MORTALITY

In this section we will consider gender differences in both mortality and morbidity and the reasons that have been put forward to explain these. Firstly, if we look at life expectancy we find that in most parts of the world women live longer than men. In the period 2017–2019, life expectancy at birth in the UK was 79.4 for men and 83.1 for women. In 2020, life expectancy at birth had declined to 78.6 years for men and 82.6 years for women. This decline was believed to be due to the COVID-19 pandemic but it is unclear whether or how quickly life expectancy will improve post-pandemic. The UK was already falling behind other European countries in terms of life expectancy (ONS, 2022a). There is thus a gap of between 3 and 4 years in life expectancy at birth between men and women in the UK (King's Fund, 2022). We should note however that this is largely a phenomenon of more affluent countries. In some poorer countries the life expectancy gap between men and women is negligible. Furthermore, we should remember the impact of other intersecting factors, such as class and race so that, for example, a middle class professional man is likely to outlive most women who are less privileged (Bergeron-Boucher et al., 2022).

Various explanations have been suggested for this difference in life expectancy. One explanation is that women have a biological advantage which protects them from early death from cardiovascular disease, since female sex hormones can to some extent protect women from cardiovascular disease prior to the menopause. However, this assumption has in the past led to heart disease being under diagnosed in women and as a result women who do have heart disease have a higher death rate than men (Hobson & Bakker, 2019).

The most important explanation for gender differences in mortality is health behaviours. Until recently, men's uptake of smoking was considerably higher than women's. The gap between smoking rates for men and women has narrowed as smoking rates have fallen, however, men's smoking rate is still higher. In 2021, 15.1% of men and 11.5% of women were current smokers. This was the lowest level of smoking on record (ONS, 2022b). Since smoking rates were higher and the gender gap was much wider in the past, it is likely that amongst older generations there will still be considerably more men than women who are either current or ex-smokers. Other differences in health behaviours also contribute to the difference in mortality rates with men more likely to engage in a range of risky behaviours, such as heavy drinking and dangerous driving. Men thus have higher rates of accidental death and deaths from homicide. Men also have alcohol-related and drug misuse–related death rates that are double those among women and substantially higher rates of suicide (Dobson, 2006).

The Australian sociologist, Connell, produced a theory describing what she called the **'gender order'**. This theory can help to explain these differences in mortality. Connell described the gender order as a set of institutional structures which allowed one gender (men) to dominate the other (women) (Connell, 2009). The gender order produces a set of social arrangements which perpetuate inequalities between men and women in how work is organised; where power is held and how these power differences translate into intimate and sexual relationships. Thus, Connell suggests, that gender identities (i.e. what counts as acceptable masculine and feminine behaviours and identities) are not biologically determined but culturally formed and it is these identities that perpetuate the gender order. Connell identifies four types of masculinity which she calls **hegemonic, complicit, subordinate** and **marginalised**. Although other types of masculinity were described by Connell, she believed that hegemonic masculinity was the dominant form so it is the focus of this discussion.

The label **'hegemonic masculinity'** comes from the Greek word 'hegemony' which means the dominance of one social group over another. Thus, Connell is saying that hegemonic masculinity is that form of masculinity that promotes the dominance of men in society (Connell & Messerschmidt, 2005). Connell also described the dominant cultural form of femininity as 'emphasised femininity'. She argues that the gender order idealises of the woman who expends energy on her appearance to make herself attractive and desirable to men. The other traits of the ideal woman emphasised within the gender order include compliance, subordination to the needs of men, empathy, nurturance and sensitivity. However, despite these traits being idealised within the gender order, emphasised femininity is treated as being inferior to masculinity.

Typical values associated with hegemonic masculinity include physical toughness and aggression, risk taking, competitiveness and an inability to admit weakness or dependence on others. Hegemonic masculinity is promoted in the media through products, such as computer games, violent action movies and men's magazines. There is evidence to support the argument that this traditional form of masculinity has contributed to health behaviours that are damaging to men's health. This is firstly due to increased risk taking and secondly to the fact that men may see asking for help as a form of weakness and thus delay seeking medical advice (Evans et al., 2011).

Masculinity may intersect with other factors, such as age and occupation, for example, road accident deaths are more common in young men. Traditionally, many men worked in dangerous and health-damaging industries, such as coal mining where physical toughness was a required attribute. However, these traditional work patterns have changed as many of these industries have declined. However, although we noted earlier that gender roles and identities are becoming more fluid, hegemonic masculinity still has a dominant place in contemporary culture. Connell argues that the gender order can be damaging for both men and women. Hegemonic masculinity justifies gender inequality and exposes women to everyday sexism and male violence but it damages men's health too. The damaging impacts of hegemonic masculinity on men's health corroborate this (Connell, 2009). Given the negative impacts of hegemonic masculinity on men's health, (Evans et al., 2011) suggest that it should be considered as an additional social determinant of ill health in men.

GENDER DIFFERENCES IN MORBIDITY

We have said that women have an average life expectancy which is a few years higher than that of men. This can mainly be explained by differences in health behaviours. However, women have traditionally reported significantly poorer health than men. This has been described as the 'gender paradox', that is, although women are sicker, it is men who die sooner. One hypothesis has been that men tend to under report health problems while women are more willing to admit to them. This gap in self-reported ill health between men and women has been narrowing. Recent studies have suggested a much more complex, intersecting pattern of gender differences in health, since factors such as age, race and social class all have an impact on these differences. However, a large number of studies have continued to point to higher levels of morbidity among women, particularly in less affluent countries (Sen et al., 2007).

In a report to the World Health Organization, Sen et al. (2007) suggested that higher levels of morbidity among women can be attributed to a mix of biological sex differences and gendered social determinants. Biological sex differences mainly relate to ill health linked to reproduction, for example, complications of childbirth or reproductive cancers, such as breast and cervical cancer. Gendered social determinants that affect women's health include poorer pay and working conditions, a higher burden of unpaid work in the home and gender-based violence. Thus, the requirements of 'emphasised femininity' can place heavy burdens on women and reduce their autonomy and ability to control their own health.

The requirements of emphasised femininity can also place a toll on women's health in respect of the burden of living up to the idealised images of femininity projected in the mass media. Anorexia and other eating disorders are conditions mainly, but not exclusively, experienced by women and are associated with a negative body image, a fear of being fat and a subjective sense of powerlessness (Rich, 2006). Anorexia is one of the most fatal of psychiatric illnesses (van Hoeken

& Hoek, 2020). Saguy and Gruys (2010) suggest that the media portrays thinness in women as associated with virtue, self-control and attractiveness. By contrast, fatness is stigmatised and treated as a symbol of laziness, unattractiveness and lack of self-control. Thus, this pejorative discourse, coupled with the unrealistic, airbrushed images of models and celebrities projected in the media has led to widespread body dissatisfaction among young women. This has been thought to contribute to the rise in anorexia in contemporary society (Wykes & Gunter, 2004). We look further at body dissatisfaction and fat stigma in Chapter 5.

Women may live longer than men but do not do better than men in terms of 'healthy life expectancy' for the reasons outlined above. Many women spend a large part of their later life living with long-standing illness. Women also have higher rates of anxiety and depression in addition to their higher rates of eating disorders described above. Many of the conditions that women live with in later life are also disabling to some degree (Murtagh & Hubert, 2004). In particular, women experience more inflammatory diseases, such as arthritis and lupus; for example, 8% of the population experience some form of autoimmune disease and 80% of these are women (Criado Perez, 2019). These diseases are under-researched and some authors have suggested that women's health has often not been taken seriously. This has sometimes led to a dismissive attitude to women's higher levels of self-reported ill health in the medical literature; the implication being that women are just complainers (Cleghorn, 2021). This leads us to consider our next issue, namely the extent to which policymakers, health researchers and health professionals have or have not taken women's health seriously.

Gender Bias in Medicine and Healthcare

GENDER BIAS IN MEDICAL SCIENCES

Before considering whether there is contemporary gender bias in healthcare, we will look briefly at the history of medicine's understanding of, and attitudes towards, women's bodies. The Greek physician, Hippocrates, who was born in around 460 BC has been regarded as the 'father' of medicine. His ideas were further developed by another Greek physician called Galen who was born in 129 AD. The ideas of Hippocrates formed the foundations of medicine for almost two millennia, only being supplanted in the late 18th century 'enlightenment' period due to the rapid scientific progress and changes in philosophical ideas that occurred at that time. Two central ideas dominated medical ideas about women's bodies for many centuries. Firstly, medicine was '**androcentric**' meaning that the man was seen as the ideal version of a human being and women's bodies were valued against male standards and found to be deficient. If the male body was the norm then the female body was a faulty, smaller, weaker version lacking male sex organs (Bonnard, 2014). Criado Perez (2019) suggests that medicine is still androcentric. Medical students learn anatomy and female anatomy. The male body represents normal anatomy and the female body is presented as deviating from this (Criado Perez, 2019). Surveys of anatomy textbooks have shown that men's bodies predominate in illustrations and are still often presented as the norm (Lawrence & Bendixon, 1992). A recent study of Dutch medical textbooks showed a persistence of gender bias in medical texts (Dijkstra et al., 2008).

The second central idea of Hippocratic medicine was that women's purpose was to bear and raise children; anything which distracted them from this central purpose was bad for them and all women's diseases were caused by their reproductive system. The Greeks and many generations of doctors after them believed that the womb could 'wander' about the body, making mischief, if it was deprived of its 'natural' function which was to bear children. A huge number of illnesses were attributed to the wandering womb including breathlessness caused by 'womb suffocation' when the womb 'rose up' in the body. These medical ideas also justified the belief that women should not be educated, since women's mental activity could 'starve' the womb. The cure of many of women's illnesses was thus said by male physicians to be to fulfil their 'natural' purpose by being married young and bearing as many children as possible (Cleghorn, 2021). The idea of the womb as the source of all women's mental and physical ills persisted right into the 20th century in the diagnosis of hysteria commonly applied to women for a variety of symptoms. The term comes from the Greek word for womb, namely, hysterus. Hysteria was only removed from the official list of psychiatric diseases in 1952 (Jones, 2015). It has, however, left a legacy of prejudiced beliefs, such as that women's accounts are unreliable and emotional and that their illnesses are less serious and more likely to be psychological in origin.

Thus, a large number of historical studies have suggested that gender bias was built into medical science and practice from its earliest origins and that this bias has been very resistant to change. If we look first at androcentric bias in medicine (the idea that the male is the 'norm'), this bias has had a number of impacts on medical sciences. There has been a neglect of research into illnesses predominantly suffered by women, such as osteoporosis, endometriosis and lupus, often as a result of a lack of funding (Criado Perez, 2019). Sen et al. (2007) have suggested that there is gender bias throughout the field of health research affecting policymakers, ethical committees and research-funding bodies as well as disadvantaging women scientists. Holdcroft (2007) has suggested that gender bias in medical research means that the evidence base to medicine is fundamentally flawed. Many common well-established medicines were approved on the basis of trials mainly or exclusively conducted on men as there was an assumption that female hormones could 'interfere' with trial results. As the male was considered the norm, testing drugs on women was deemed unnecessary. Even in more recent trials, male subjects predominate. For example, a meta-analysis of 27 trials for statins showed that only 16% of the subjects were women (Holdcroft, 2007). Women have a higher rate of adverse drug reactions and this could, in some cases, be because they are taking drugs that were never tested on women (Franconi et al., 2007).

Androcentric bias has also affected sciences, such as ergonomics concerned with the health and safety of everyday technologies. Many of the tools, clothing and equipment that women use in their everyday lives, such as cars, work tools and sports equipment have been designed to fit men (Criado Perez, 2019). For example, until very recently the crash test dummies used to test car safety were based exclusively on the average male build. Only in 2022 did a Swedish company bring a female crash test dummy onto the market (BBC, 2022). This may go some way to explaining the higher rate of whiplash injury in women. Similarly, both computer keyboards and piano keyboards are designed for male hands, making women more at risk of repetitive strain injury. Much 'unisex' protective clothing used in the workplace is designed for the male torso and women may have problems of fit and comfort which compromise their health and safety (TUC, 2017). We have seen recently during the COVID-19 pandemic the risks associated with lack of attention to the provision of adequate personal protective equipment particularly to people in care work (Shelton et al., 2022). Payne and Doyal (2010) have suggested that there has been a general neglect of the specific hazards faced by women in the workforce by occupational medicine which traditionally focused on industrial hazards faced by men. The risks to older women in the workplace have been particularly neglected. Women face particular risks associated with repetitive movements, such as keyboard and assembly line work. Women in care work face risk of exposure to infection as well as the risk of exposure to violence and to injuries associated with lifting and handling people (Payne & Doyal, 2010).

GENDER BIAS IN HEALTHCARE PRACTICE

We have seen that gender bias in medical sciences has led to a neglect of women's illnesses. We look now at the legacy of beliefs about women's propensity to 'hysteria' in clinical practice. In clinical practice, a tendency to take women's symptoms less seriously than men's has been widely reported (Hamberg, 2008). Women have often reported negative experiences of healthcare, reporting that their problems have been dismissed or not taken seriously (Cleghorn, 2021). Studies of gender bias in the medical profession have to some degree validated women's complaints. Women are less likely than men to be referred for tests or referred to a specialist by GPs (Hamberg, 2008). They are more likely to find that their GP views their illness as psychogenic or 'medically unexplained' (Malterud, 2000) and they are more likely to be prescribed drugs, such as opioids and benzodiazepines (Oppenheim, 2022). They may also have to wait longer for treatment (Criado Perez, 2019). The propensity of some doctors to question the mental health of women reporting physical symptoms has been called **'medical gaslighting'** by campaigners.

MEDICAL GASLIGHTING

The term 'gaslighting' is derived from a 1938 play by Patrick Hamilton called 'Gas Light' in which a husband manipulates his wife in order to convince her that she is going insane. The term gained currency in the 21st century to describe psychological manipulation used to convince someone that they cannot trust their perception of reality. It has been described as a form of psychological abuse. The term 'medical gaslighting' has been used by both activists and some researchers to describe those occasions when women have healthcare experiences in which their physical symptoms are disbelieved and invalidated and their mental health questioned (Sebring, 2021).

Gender disparities are particularly evident in medical judgments regarding men and women's reports of pain. A number of studies have suggested that clinicians tend to underestimate pain in women and attribute it to 'emotional' causes (Samulowitz et al., 2018). A classic study of a pain clinic found that men were recorded as 'experiencing' pain, while women were recorded as 'complaining of' pain and were more likely to be described as hypochondriacs (Lack, 1982). A more recent study of an emergency department found women presenting with acute abdominal pain considerably less likely to be treated with analgesia than men (Chen et al., 2008). Similarly, there is a considerable body of evidence showing gender bias in the treatment of coronary heart disease (CHD). Women presenting with chest pain have had their pain treated less seriously than men. They are less likely to be referred to a cardiologist and more likely to be treated on a 'wait and see' basis (Liaudat et al., 2018). This may go some way to explaining the poorer survival rate of women with CHD.

Older women experience gender bias that is compounded by ageism. These biases can affect diagnoses and treatment decisions and lead to disparities in care when older women are deemed too 'frail' for aggressive treatments (Chrisler et al., 2016). A study in 2019 suggested gender bias also affects the diagnosis of frailty and recommendations for surgery (Tam et al., 2020). Since COVID-19, the diagnosis of frailty has increasingly played an important role in decisions about whether or not to offer treatment, such as surgery and critical care and thus gender bias could be life threatening for the women affected. A study in 2007 found that women over 50 are less likely to be admitted to critical care than men with the same severity of illness (Fowler et al., 2007). We will look in more detail at the intersection of ageism and gender bias in healthcare in Chapter 10.

Many illnesses that mainly affect women are associated with extremely long delays before diagnosis. For example, lupus is a multi-system, autoimmune disease mainly affecting women. In the UK, women wait over six years on average for a diagnosis and almost half are initially diagnosed with mental health problems or 'medically unexplained' symptoms (Sloan et al., 2020). Lupus can have serious complications, such as kidney failure, and diagnostic delay in lupus leads to worse outcomes (Kernder et al., 2021). Denny (2004) found that women with endometriosis also waited over six years for a diagnosis and over half of women were initially told there was nothing wrong. The majority of women thought that doctors did not take their symptoms seriously.

Case Example: 'Medical Gaslighting' and Diagnostic Delay

The author, Hilary Mantel's autobiography described her attempts to get a diagnosis for severe endometriosis in her twenties. As a university student, she was not believed and instead referred for psychiatric treatment where she was diagnosed with 'stress due to over ambition'. She was given anti-psychotic medication and then admitted to an inpatient psychiatric unit for what was presumed to be an 'imaginary' illness. She only received a correct diagnosis and surgery some years later, partly as a result of her own research into the illness. By this point the disease had caused serious organ damage which among other things prevented her from ever having children. She said of her experiences:

'Endometriosis is a gynaecological condition with a dazzling array of systemic effects. It is not rare, though mercifully it is rare for the disease to run on, unrecognised, for as long as it did in me, and it is rare for it to do such damage. Because of the number of symptoms it throws up it is sometimes hard to diagnose. It is always hard to diagnose, for a doctor who doesn't listen and doesn't look'.

(MANTEL, 2004, p. 184)

REFLECTION POINT

Think about your own experiences of healthcare and whether you have seen or experienced gender bias either as a patient or as a member of staff. How do you think that gender bias might affect the patients experiencing it? What do you think should be done to tackle gender bias in the health sciences and in clinical care?

The UK Department of Health and Social Care published a Women's Health Strategy for England in 2022 (DHSC, 2022). This acknowledged that women suffered higher levels of morbidity than men and that the 'male as default' model had led to deficiencies in women's care and treatment. It also acknowledged that women's voices had often been ignored by health professionals and policymakers. The strategy aimed to give women more say in their care and to boost women's representation in healthcare decision making. So far, there is limited evidence of implementation.

WOMEN, MEDICINE AND CHILDBIRTH

For many women, their first prolonged contact with health services will be during pregnancy and childbirth. Oakley (2016) suggests that childbirth is the transition for many women into the role of motherhood which all too often has also marked the point where their lives became increasingly circumscribed by gender inequalities. Unfortunately, childbirth also too often marked a point where women first felt that control of their bodies was taken from them by an unresponsive healthcare system (DHSC, 2022). There has been a marked change in the management of childbirth in the post-war era. In the 1940s and 1950s, most births took place at home. By the twenty-first century, however, over 95% of births took place in hospital. Sociologists, such as Oakley (2016), described an increasing cascade of medical interventions in childbirth with rates of medical induction of labour, episiotomy, instrumental delivery and caesarean sections all going up over this period. Sociologists began to question whether this rise in interventions was really driven by clinical need. For example, a classic study of childbirth by Cartwright (1979) showed that administrative factors were the main drivers of artificial induction of labour as opposed to clear clinical reasons for this intervention. Childbirth had become increasingly medicalised and was governed by a risk discourse which justified increasing levels of medical interference in the process of labour (Scamell, 2014).

In reaction to this, a movement advocating a return to 'natural' childbirth and home births developed from the 1970s onwards spearheaded by pressure groups, such as the National Childbirth Trust. These groups advocated a more 'natural' approach to childbirth; questioned the efficacy and safety of much medical intervention and advocated a return to home births with minimal medical intervention. They were highly critical of the 'medical model' of childbirth arguing that birth was a normal physiological process (van Teijlingen, 2005). The argument between those advocating medicalised childbirth with increased use of technological interventions to 'manage' birth and those advocating 'natural' childbirth have at times become polarised in ways that can be bewildering for pregnant women (Oakley, 2016). For women, the most important issue is the opportunity to be listened to and to make an informed choice which best meets their personal and clinical circumstances (DHSC, 2022). It is important to remember that women's social circumstances have an important bearing on the choices they feel able to make. It is often socioeconomic and cultural factors that have the most important impact on both women's experiences of pregnancy and childbirth and its outcomes (WHO, 2018).

Sexual and Gender Minorities and Health Inequalities

There has recently been greater focus on inequalities in the health of sexual and gender minorities. SGM, such as lesbian, gay and transgender people can suffer disadvantages, stigma and discrimination that can adversely affect their health. Differences in health behaviours among SGM sub groups, such as men who have sex with men (MSM), may also impact on health. There are considerable gaps in our knowledge of the health of sexual and gender minorities and much of the evidence that we do have is poor quality. However, we do know that SGM have poor self-reported health and higher levels of mental ill health (Blondeel et al., 2016; WHO, 2016). Rates of suicide and self-harm, anxiety, depression and substance misuse have all been found to be higher in SGM (McDermott et al., 2021).

Among MSM and transgender people there is also a higher prevalence of HIV infection globally, though this varies widely between countries with prevalence rates being highest in the Caribbean and Sub-Saharan Africa (Blondeel et al., 2016). Higher rates of other sexually transmitted infections, such as syphilis, hepatitis and human papillomavirus (HPV) have all been found in MSM and transgender people and this higher rate of sexually transmitted infections has been linked to risk behaviours (Blondeel et al., 2016). The WHO suggests that these risk behaviours are highest in settings where SGM face marginalisation, stigma and violence (WHO, 2016). A number of studies have shown that SGM are at higher risk of violence and victimisation particularly homophobic violence. There is also some evidence that MSM are also at higher risk of intimate partner violence (Blondeel et al., 2016).

There is evidence that SGM have more difficulties engaging with health services with a significant minority (38%) reporting negative experiences because of their gender identity. A number of problems have been reported including SGM experiencing discriminatory attitudes and language from staff, a lack of care tailored to the needs of SGM and an environment that is not conducive to SGM disclosing their gender identity (Government Equalities Office, 2018). Some studies have reported that SGM have had less positive experiences of cancer care which alienated them from psychosocial support services (Fish & Williamson, 2018; Hulbert-Williams et al., 2017). Older SGM are more likely to be living alone and to lack social support making sympathetic health and social care services an even more important source of support (Bolderston & Ralph, 2016). This group may have grown up in an era when homosexuality was illegal and some will have lived a largely 'closeted' life making disclosure of sexual orientation or gender identity more difficult (Fish & Karben, 2015).

Varney suggests that we need to increase efforts to provide inclusive 'rainbow medicine' which is sensitive to the needs of SGM (Varney, 2016). This should include addressing stigmatising attitudes among health and social care staff and creating a welcoming and SGM-friendly environment where SGM can feel safe to disclose their identity. We also need to educate staff to better understand and provide for the specific health needs of SGM (Bolderston & Ralph, 2016). Unfortunately, a recent survey showed that 72% of care staff had had no training in SGM health, so much still needs to be done to create equitable, inclusive and welcoming health services for sexual and gender minorities (Varney, 2016).

REFLECTION POINT

What practical steps do you think health services could take to create a welcoming environment for people from sexual and gender minorities? How confident or otherwise are you that the current healthcare system can provide inclusive and equitable care for this group of people? If you are not confident, then what needs to change?

Summary of Key Points

- Many sociologists see gender identity as socially constructed rather than biologically determined.
- Despite some improvements in the rights of women, gender inequality remains ingrained in society.
- Men in the UK have a lower life expectancy than women. This has been linked to health behaviours which have, in turn, been linked to a culture of 'hegemonic masculinity'.
- Women have a higher rate of morbidity. This can be linked to women's experience of social disadvantage, everyday sexism and discrimination.
- There is evidence of gender bias in medical sciences which can have negative impacts on women's treatment and care.
- Many women have experienced gender bias in clinical care. This can negatively affect both health outcomes and their experience of care.
- Sexual and gender minorities have frequently reported experiencing discrimination and stigma which negatively affected their health and experiences of healthcare.

Further Reading

Cleghorn, E (2022). *Unwell women: Misdiagnosis and myth in a man-made world*. Penguin.
Criado Perez, C (2019). *Invisible women*. Penguin Books.
Evans, M (2017). *The Persistence of gender inequality*. Polity Press.
Varney, J (2016). Rainbow medicine–supporting the needs of lesbian, gay, bisexual and trans patients. *Clinical Medicine, 16*(5), 405.

References

Age UK. (2021). *Pensioner Poverty*. Retrieved February 19, 2023, from. https://www.ageuk.org.uk/globalassets/age-uk/documents/annual-reports-and-reviews/age-uk-pensioner-poverty-report.pdf.
Annandale, E., & Hunt, K. (Eds.). (2000). *Gender inequalities in health*. Open University Press.
Annesley, C, & Bennett, F (2011). Universal Credit may reinforce the traditional 'male breadwinner' model and affect many women's access to an income. *British Politics and Policy at LSE*. http://blogs.lse.ac.uk/politicsandpolicy/2011/06/21/universal-credit-inequality/.
Bates, L. (2016). *Everyday sexism*. Simon and Schuster.
BBC (2022). The crash test dummy aimed at protecting women drivers. Retrieved December 6, 2023, from https://www.bbc.co.uk/news/technology-62877930.
Bergeron-Boucher, M. P., Alvarez, J. A., Kashnitsky, I., & Zarulli, V. (2022). Probability of males to outlive females: An international comparison from 1751 to 2020. *BMJ Open, 12*(8), e059964.

Blondeel, K, Say, L, Chou, D, Toskin, I, Khosla, R, Scolaro, E, & Temmerman, M. (2016). Evidence and knowledge gaps on the disease burden in sexual and gender minorities: A review of systematic reviews. *International Journal for Equity in Health, 15*(1), 1–9.

Bolderston, A, & Ralph, S. (2016). Improving the health care experiences of lesbian, gay, bisexual and transgender patients. *Radiography, 22*(3), 207–211.

Bonnard, J. B., (2014). Male and female bodies according to Ancient Greek physicians. *Clio Women, Gender, History*(37).

Bryson, V. (2016). *Feminist political theory.* Bloomsbury Publishing.

Bryson, V. (2021). *The Futures of Feminism.* Manchester University Press.

Buchanan, I, Pratt, I, & Francis-Devine, B. (2023). *Women and the UK economy. Research Briefing, 6838.* House of Commons Library. https://researchbriefings.files.parliament.uk/documents/SN06838/SN06838.pdf.

Carpenter, M. (2000). Reinforcing the pillars: Rethinking gender, social divisions and health. In E. Annandale, & K. Hunt. (Eds.), *Gender inequalities in health* (pp. 36–63). Open University Press.

Cartwright, A. (1979). *The dignity of labour?* Tavistock.

Chen, E. H., Shofer, F. S., Dean, A. J., Hollander, J. E., Baxt, W. G., Robey, J. L., Sease, K. L., & Mills, A. M. (2008). Gender disparity in analgesic treatment of emergency department patients with acute abdominal pain. *Academic Emergency Medicine, 15*(5), 414–418.

Chrisler, J C, Barney, A, & Palatino, B (2016). Ageism can be hazardous to women's health: Ageism, sexism, and stereotypes of older women in the healthcare system. *Journal of Social Issues, 72*(1), 86–104.

Cleghorn, E. (2021). *Unwell women: Misdiagnosis and myth in a man-made world.* Penguin Books.

Connell, R. (2009). *Gender.* Polity Press.

Connell, R. W., & Messerschmidt, J. W., (2005). Hegemonic masculinity: Rethinking the concept. *Gender & Society, 19*(6), 829–859.

Crenshaw, K. W., (2017). *On intersectionality: Essential writings.* The New Press.

Criado Perez, C. (2019). *Invisible women.* Penguin Books.

Denny, E. (2004). Women's experience of endometriosis. *Journal of Advanced Nursing, 46*(6), 641–648.

Department of Health and Social Care (DHSC). (2022). *Women's Health Strategy for England.* Retrieved December 6, 2023, from. https://www.gov.uk/government/publications/womens-health-strategy-for-england/womens-health-strategy-for-england.

Dijkstra, A. F., Verdonk, P, & Lagro-Janssen, A. L., (2008). Gender bias in medical textbooks: Examples from coronary heart disease, depression, alcohol abuse and pharmacology. *Medical Education, 42*(10), 1021–1028.

Dobson, R. (2006). Men are more likely than women to die early. *BMJ, 333*(7561), 220.

Evans, J, Frank, B, Oliffe, J. L., & Gregory, D. (2011). Health, illness, men and masculinities (HIMM): A theoretical framework for understanding men and their health. *Journal of Men's Health, 8*(1), 7–15.

Evans, M. (2017). *The persistence of gender inequality.* Polity Press.

Fawcett Society (2019). The gender pay gap and pay discrimination—Explainer. https://www.fawcettsociety.org.uk/the-gender-pay-gap-and-pay-discrimination-explainer

Fish, J, & Williamson, I. (2018). Exploring lesbian, gay and bisexual patients' accounts of their experiences of cancer care in the UK. *European Journal of Cancer Care, 27*(1), 12501.

Fish, J, & Karban, K. (Eds.). (2015). *Lesbian, gay, bisexual and trans health inequalities.* Policy Press.

Fowler, R A, Sabur, N, Li, P, Juurlink, D. N., Pinto, R, Hladunewich, M. A., Adhikari, N. K., Sibbald, W. J., & Martin, C. M. (2007). Sex-and age-based differences in the delivery and outcomes of critical care. *CMAJ, 177*(12), 1513–1519.

Franconi, F, Brunelleschi, S, Steardo, L, & Cuomo, V. (2007). Gender differences in drug responses. *Pharmacological Research, 55*(2), 81–95.

Giddens, A., & Sutton, P. W. (2017). *Sociology.* Polity Press.

Gkiouleka, A, Huijts, T, Beckfield, J, & Bambra, C. (2018). Understanding the micro and macro politics of health: Inequalities, intersectionality & institutions—A research agenda. *Social Science & Medicine, 200*, 92–98.

Government Equalities Office. (2018). *LGBT action plan: Improving the lives of lesbian, gay, bisexual and transgender people.* Retrieved Janury 2, 2023, from. https://assets.publishing.service.gov.uk/media/5b39e91ee5274a0bbef01fd5/GEO-LGBT-Action-Plan.pdf.

Government Equalities Office. (2019). *Variations in sex characteristics: Technical paper.* Retrieved December 6, 2023, from. https://assets.publishing.service.gov.uk/government/uploads/system/uploads/attachment_data/file/771468/VSC_Technical_Paper_Web_Accessible.pdf.

Hamberg, K. (2008). Gender bias in medicine. *Women's Health, 4*(3), 237–243.

Hobson, P, & Bakker, J. (2019). How the heart attack gender gap is costing women's lives. *British Journal of Cardiac Nursing, 14*(11), 1–3.

Holdcroft, A. (2007). Gender bias in research: How does it affect evidence based medicine? *Journal of the Royal Society of Medicine, 100*(1), 2–3.

Hulbert-Williams, N. J., Plumpton, C. O., Flowers, P, McHugh, R, Neal, R. D., & Semlyen J & Storey, L. (2017). The cancer care experiences of gay, lesbian and bisexual patients: A secondary analysis of data from the UK Cancer Patient Experience Survey. *European Journal of Cancer Care, 26*(4), 12670.

Institute of Fiscal Studies. (2021). *Gender differences in subject choice leads to gender pay gap immediately after graduation.* Retrieved December 6, 2023, from. https://ifs.org.uk/articles/gender-differences-subject-choice-leads-gender-pay-gap-immediately-after-graduation.

Johnson, A. H. (2019). Rejecting, reframing, and reintroducing: Trans people's strategic engagement with the medicalisation of gender dysphoria. *Sociology of Health & Illness, 41*(3), 517–532.

Jones, C. E. (2015). Wandering wombs and "female troubles": The hysterical origins, symptoms, and treatments of endometriosis. *Women's Studies, 44*(8), 1083–1113.

Kernder, A, Richter, J G, Fischer-Betz, R, Winkler-Rohlfing, B, Brinks, R, Aringer, M, & Chehab, G. (2021). Delayed diagnosis adversely affects outcome in systemic lupus erythematosus: Cross sectional analysis of the LuLa cohort. *Lupus, 30*(3), 431–438.

King's Fund. (2022). *What is Happening to Life Expectancy in England?* Retrieved December 6, 2023, from. https://www.kingsfund.org.uk/publications/whats-happening-life-expectancy-england?gclid=EAIaIQobChMIgoyUk4Kz_QIVnoBQBh2RvgbCEAAYAyAAEgJDHPD_BwE.

Lack, D. Z. (1982). Women and pain: Another feminist issue. *Women & Therapy, 1*(1), 55–64.

Lawrence, S. C., & Bendixen, K. (1992). His and hers: Male and female anatomy in anatomy texts for US medical students, 1890–1989. *Social Science & Medicine, 35*(7), 925–934.

Liaudat, C, Vaucher, P, De Francesco, T, Jaunin-Stalder, N, Herzig, L, & Verdon F & Clair, C. (2018). Sex/gender bias in the management of chest pain in ambulatory care. *Women's health, 14*, 1–9.

Maddock Jones R. (2022). Just 4% of FTSE 350 CEOs are women investment week. Retrieved December 6, 2023, from https://www.investmentweek.co.uk/news/4057425/ftse-350-ceos-women.

Malterud, K. (2000). Symptoms as a source of medical knowledge: Understanding medically unexplained disorders in women. *Family Medicine, 32*(9), 603–611.

Mantel, H. (2004). *Giving up the ghost: A memoir.* Henry Holt and Company.

McDermott, E, Nelson, R, & Weeks, H. (2021). The politics of LGBT+ health inequality: Conclusions from a UK scoping review. *International Journal of Environmental Research and Public Health, 18*(2), 826.

Miller, E. M., & Costello, C. Y. (2001). The limits of biological determinism. *American Sociological Review, 66*(4), 592–598.

Murtagh, K. N., & Hubert, H. B. (2004). Gender differences in physical disability among an elderly cohort. *American Journal of Public Health, 94*(8), 1406–1411.

Oakley, A. (2016). The sociology of childbirth: An autobiographical journey through four decades of research. *Sociology of Health & Illness, 38*(5), 689–705.

Office of National Statistics (ONS). (2022). *Mortality in England and Wales: Past and projected trends in average lifespan.* Retrieved January 2, 2024, from. https://www.ons.gov.uk/peoplepopulationandcommunity/birthsdeathsandmarriages/lifeexpectancies/articles/mortalityinenglandandwales/pastandprojectedtrendsinaveragelifespan#:~:text=1.,(COVID%2D19)%20pandemic.

O'Neil, A, Sojo, V, Fileborn, B, Scovelle, A J, & Milner, A. (2018). The# MeToo movement: An opportunity in public health? *The Lancet, 391*(10140), 2587–2589.

ONS. (2022). *Adult smoking rates in the UK.* Retrieved January 2, 2024, from. https://www.ons.gov.uk/peoplepopulationandcommunity/healthandsocialcare/healthandlifeexpectancies/bulletins/adultsmokinghabitsingreatbritain/2021#:~:text=Across%20all%20constituent%20countries%20of,million)%20reported%20being%20current%20smokers.

Oppenheim, M. (2022). Hundreds of thousands more women than men prescribed powerful anti-anxiety drugs 'harder to come off than heroin. *The Independent.* Retrieved March 6, 2023, from. https://www.independent.co.uk/news/uk/home-news/benzodiazepines-more-women-prescribed-than-men-b2184230.html.

Oxford Dictionary of Biography. (2004). Blake, Sophia Louisa Jex. https://www.oxforddnb.com/display/10.1093/ref:odnb/9780198614128.001.0001/odnb-9780198614128-e-34189

Payne, S, & Doyal, L. (2010). Older women, work and health. *Occupational Medicine, 60*(3), 172–177.

Prout, A. (1986). Wet children' and 'little actresses': Going sick in primary school. *Sociology of Health & Illness, 8*(2), 113–136.

Rich, E. (2006). Anorexic dis (connection): Managing anorexia as an illness and an identity. *Sociology of Health & Illness, 28*(3), 284–305.

Saguy, A. C., & Gruys, K. (2010). Morality and health: News media constructions of overweight and eating disorders. *Social Problems, 57*(2), 231–250.

Salem, S. (2018). Intersectionality and its discontents: Intersectionality as traveling theory. *European Journal of Women's Studies, 25*(4), 403–418.

Samulowitz, A, Gremyr, I, Eriksson, E, & Hensing, G. (2018). Brave men" and "emotional women": A theory-guided literature review on gender bias in health care and gendered norms towards patients with chronic pain. *Pain Research and Management, 2018*, 6358624.

Scamell, M. (2014). Childbirth within the Risk Society. *Sociology Compass, 8*(7), 917–928.

Sebring, J. C. (2021). Towards a sociological understanding of medical gaslighting in western health care. *Sociology of Health & Illness, 43*(9), 1951–1964.

Sen, G, Östlin, P, & George, A. (2007). *Unequal, unfair, ineffective and inefficient: Gender inequity in health; why it exists and how we can change it. Final Report to the WHO Commission on Social Determinants of Health, Women and Gender Equity Knowledge Network*. World Health Organisation.

Shelton, C, El-Boghdadly, K, & Appleby, J. B. (2022). The 'haves' and 'have-nots' of personal protective equipment during the COVID-19 pandemic: The ethics of emerging inequalities amongst healthcare workers. *Journal of Medical Ethics, 48*(10), 653–657.

Shifrer, D, & Frederick, A. (2019). Disability at the intersections. *Sociology Compass, 13*(10), 12733.

Skills for Care. (2010). *The state of the adult social care workforce in England*. Skills for Care.

Sloan, M, Harwood, R, Sutton, S, D'Cruz, D, Howard, P, Wincup, C, Brimicombe, J, & Gordon, C. (2020). Medically explained symptoms: A mixed methods study of diagnostic, symptom and support experiences of patients with lupus and related systemic autoimmune diseases. *Rheumatology Advances in Practice, 4*(1), rkaa006.

Smith, V. (2023). *Hags: The demonisation of middle aged women*. Little Brown Book Group.

Statista (2023). Gender pay gap for median gross hourly earnings in the United Kingdom from 1997 to 2023. Retrieved December 6, 2023, from https://www.statista.com/statistics/280710/uk-gender-pay-gap/.

Tam, V, Tong, B, Gorawara-Bhat, R, Liao, C, & Ferguson, M. K. (2020). Gender bias affects assessment of frailty and recommendations for surgery. *The Annals of Thoracic Surgery, 109*(3), 938–944.

The Everyday Sexism Project (2023). Retrieved December 5, 2023, from https://everydaysexism.com/.

Trade Union Congress (TUC) (2017). *Personal protective equipment and women*. https://www.tuc.org.uk/sites/default/files/PPEandwomenguidance.pdf

van Hoeken, D, & Hoek, HW. (2020). Review of the burden of eating disorders: Mortality, disability, costs, quality of life, and family burden. *Current Opinion in Psychiatry, 33*(6), 521–527.

van Teijlingen, E. (2005). A critical analysis of the medical model as used in the study of pregnancy and childbirth. *Sociological Research Online, 10*(2), http://www.socresonline.org.uk/10/2/teijlingen.html.

Varney, J. (2016). Rainbow medicine—supporting the needs of lesbian, gay, bisexual and trans patients. *Clinical Medicine, 16*(5), 405.

WHO. (2016). *FAQ on health and sexual diversity—An introduction to key concepts*. World Health Organization.

WHO. (2018). Making childbirth a positive experience. Retrieved December 6, 2023, from https://www.who.int/news/item/15-02-2018-making-childbirth-a-positive-experience.

WHO. (2021) Violence against women: Prevalence estimates2018. Retrieved December 5, 2023, from. https://www.who.int/publications/i/item/9789240022256.

WHO. (2021). *Factsheet: Violence against women*. Retrieved January 2, 2024, from. https://www.who.int/news-room/fact-sheets/detail/violence-against-women.

Wollstonecraft, M. (2004). *A vindication of the rights of woman*. Penguin Books.

World Economic Forum (2020). As the UK publishes its first census of women killed by men, here's a global look at the problem. Retrieved March 9, 2023, from https://www.weforum.org/agenda/2020/11/violence-against-women-femicide-census/.

Wykes, M, & Gunter, B. (2004). The media and body image: If looks could kill. Sage Publications.

Ethnicity, 'Race' and Inequalities of Health

This chapter considers inequalities of health related to ethnicity. The causes of these inequalities include both the experience of deprivation (discussed in Chapter 2) and more specific experiences of racism and discrimination. Racism and discrimination help to create the higher rates of social deprivation found amongst many ethnic minority groups. As we discussed in Chapter 3, ethnic inequalities can intersect with other types of inequality.

To put ethnic inequalities in health into context, the chapter first reviews changing concepts of ethnicity and 'race' before looking at the particular forms of disadvantage and discrimination that can be faced by members of ethnic minority groups. It then looks at the evidence demonstrating ethnic inequalities of health. Finally, it considers whether people from ethnic minority backgrounds have equitable treatment within health services. Here, it examines whether discrimination and institutional racism worsen the care experiences of people from ethnic minority backgrounds.

Ethnicity, Race and Racism

ETHNICITY

The term 'ethnicity' is now preferred as the most accurate description of groups with different national origins and cultural backgrounds. Ethnicity tells us about the social identity of individuals and is often measured on the basis of how individuals choose to identify themselves. It denotes what Giddens and Sutton (2017) call an 'imagined community'; in other words, it is the group that people subjectively see themselves belonging to. It is important to remember that we all belong to an ethnic group, so we should not use this term only to refer to people from ethnic minority groups. Ethnic groups may have a shared history, culture, religion and shared customs. A person's ethnic identity may intersect with other aspects of their identity, such as age, class, disability and gender. This chapter uses the terminology recommended by the UK government to talk about ethnicity (Cabinet Office, 2021).

RACE

Firstly, we need to note that there is no scientific evidence to support the idea of race as a concept which describes biological differences between people from different ethnic backgrounds. Race is a social construct that operates as a political category and has been used historically to maintain the power of one group over another (Golash-Boza, 2016). The concept of race began to develop from the sixteenth century onwards for political and social reasons. The idea that separate, biologically different 'races' could be identified by skin colour and that the 'White' race was morally and intellectually superior to 'Black' or 'Oriental' races started to develop at this time but was more fully developed in the early nineteenth century (Solomos, 2003). Two key reasons were colonialism and rising European involvement in the slave trade. The idea that 'Black' or 'Oriental' races were inferior was used to justify their conquest by European colonial powers keen to plunder the natural riches of Africa and Asia (Said, 1978). At the same time, the propagation of the idea that the 'Black' races were a lesser form of humanity allowed and justified the brutality of the slave trade which treated human beings as property that could be bought and sold in the same way as cattle and other 'livestock' (Sanghera, 2021).

With the discovery of DNA and developments in our understanding of genetics, we can now say with considerable certainty that there are no clear genetic differences between these supposed 'racial' groups and that there is more diversity within ethnic groups than between them. Nowadays, more and more people have the means to investigate what their DNA tells them about their ancestry. As a result, we are all beginning to learn that we are likely to have a mixed genetic heritage. Racial theories are not only inaccurate, they are also deeply divisive. During the twentieth century, there were a number of political movements that attempted to build regimes based on racial supremacy leading to a great deal of suffering and bloodshed; in particular, Nazism in Germany and the creation of the apartheid regime by the White minority government in South Africa. Similarly, in the United States, the concept of race was used to justify racial violence conducted by White supremacist groups, such as the Ku Klux Klan. Thus, in an attempt to combat political projects based on an ideology of racial supremacy and racial violence, the UNESCO declaration on Race and Racial Prejudice in 1978 stated:

'All human beings belong to a single species and are descended from a common stock. They are born equal in dignity and rights and all form an integral part of humanity. Any theory which involves the claim that racial or ethnic groups are inherently superior or inferior, thus implying that some would be entitled to dominate or eliminate others, presumed to be inferior, or which bases value judgments on racial differentiation, has no scientific foundation and is contrary to the moral and ethical principles of humanity.'

(UNESCO, 1978)

To conclude, we talk about 'race' not to describe particular ethnic groups but in order to talk about the experience of racism and discrimination. Racist ideas within our culture originate from an unscientific ideology of racial supremacy. However outdated and inaccurate this ideology is, it still has real consequences for people from ethnic minority groups.

Racism

Racism involves a set of negative attitudes towards another ethnic group and can involve prejudice, stigma and stereotyping. Racism can take a number of forms. At an individual level, greater diversity and rising educational levels in the UK have led to greater racial tolerance and more contact between ethnic groups (Storm et al., 2017). However, there is still persistent prejudice amongst a minority of individuals. Thus, around one-quarter of the UK population are willing to describe themselves as racially prejudiced to some extent in attitude surveys. Men are more likely than women to be willing to describe themselves as racist. Recent social and political changes, such as the rise of social media and the Brexit referendum, may have increased these levels of prejudice, since some political parties and movements are more than willing to woo racially prejudiced voters (Shankley & Rhodes, 2020). Prejudice against Muslims, in particular, is more prevalent than against other minority groups, and a focus on religion rather than ethnicity is sometimes used as a political tactic to evade race discrimination legislation (Storm et al., 2020).

At an interpersonal level, these individual prejudices may be expressed through acts of aggression, bullying, abuse, violence and discrimination. On a day-to-day basis, people from ethnic minorities may experience exposure to individual acts of bigotry in the form of harassment, stereotyping, racist language and racist abuse. In one survey, more than one in eight people from ethnic minorities in the UK reported experiencing racial harassment in the past 12 months (Nazroo, 2003). Golash-Boza (2016) uses the term **'micro-aggressions'** to describe these daily insults suggesting that over time they can take a toll on the psychological well being of people from ethnic minorities. Golash-Boza (2016) suggests that racism can also be 'aversive', that is, people may avoid people who they see as different from them. This can lead to discrimination, particularly in workplaces, if people prefer to employ people who they see as similar to themselves.

Individual acts of racism can also contribute to racist bias in institutions with people from ethnic minority groups being more likely to be denied access to leisure spaces, such as restaurants, pubs and clubs. People from ethnic minorities can also be exposed to acts of violence. Racial discrimination and the promotion of racial hatred have been illegal in the UK for almost 60 years since the Race Relations Act was first passed in 1965. Race discrimination is now prohibited by the Equality Act of 2010 which also covers harassment and victimisation. Unfortunately, however, in the UK, racially motivated hate crimes have been increasing steadily since 2013 (Shankley & Rhodes, 2020). Racism is, however, not just a matter of individual prejudices and the actions arising from these. Racism can also be seen as institutional and structural. **Institutional racism** was first described in detail in the inquiry following the death of Steven Lawrence in 1993.

Case Example: Institutional Racism

Steven Lawrence was a Black British teenager killed by a gang of six White youths in an unprovoked and racially motivated attack while he was waiting for a bus. His attackers had been involved in previous racist attacks, but the police failed to arrest or charge the attackers or properly collect evidence. They instead put Steven Lawrence's family under surveillance in an attempt to discredit their attempts to get justice for their son. Steven's parents tried to bring a private prosecution in 1994, but without police cooperation the prosecution failed. Two of the attackers were finally convicted of murder in 2012 after a cold case review, but the remaining four attackers have never been brought to justice. A public inquiry in 1998–1999 found that the failure to convict the murderers of Steven Lawrence was due to the fact that the Metropolitan Police was 'institutionally racist.'

(MACPHERSON, 1999)

INSTITUTIONAL RACISM

The Macpherson inquiry (1999) into the death of Steven Lawrence defined institutional racism as 'The collective failure of an organisation to provide an appropriate and professional service to people because of their colour, culture or ethnic origin. It can be seen or detected in processes, attitudes and behaviour which amount to discrimination through unwitting prejudice, ignorance, thoughtlessness and racist stereotyping which disadvantage minority ethnic people' (MacPherson, 1999, p. 6.34).

Golash-Boza (2016) suggests that institutional (or structural) racism is built into the power structures of organisations and is hard to shift. It operates cumulatively and is often covert. Firstly, it entails turning a blind eye to individual acts of racism; for example, in a hospital ward setting, this could involve ignoring the racist abuse of a patient by another patient. Secondly, structural racism involves the perpetuation of systemic racial bias and inequality, for example in the recruitment of staff or allocation of resources. In institutionally racist organisations, long-standing policies, procedures, cultures and customs have come to privilege one ethnic group over another. The institutionally racist organisation is resistant to systemic change preferring to blame a few individual 'bad apples' when challenged over racism within the organisation. Thus, in 2023, the Casey Review identified the Metropolitan Police as still institutionally racist 30 years after the death of Steven Lawrence. It had clearly not responded adequately to the findings of the McPherson Report. It was also found to be institutionally sexist and homophobic, so we can see that a cluster of intersecting prejudices are ingrained within the organisation's culture (Casey, 2023). We will consider examples of institutional racism in healthcare at the end of this chapter.

Recently, there has been increased attention paid to individual racism (the 'bad apple' model) often at the expense of a focus on structural and institutional racism (Bourne, 2019). This has been in the form of initiatives which aim to address 'implicit' or 'unconscious' bias through activities such as training and psychological testing. Bias is framed as an individual, subconscious problem. While it is clearly a good thing to reflect critically on our biases, this approach has some weaknesses. In particular, it ignores the political, social and cultural roots of racism, and this can have unfortunate consequences (Bourne, 2019). Firstly, by framing bias as 'implicit' or 'unconscious', it can minimise individual accountability. As we have seen, racism may be conscious, with around one-quarter of the population admitting to racial prejudice in attitude surveys. We should hold people to account when these attitudes are expressed or acted upon in the workplace. Secondly, a focus on 'unconscious' bias deflects attention away from institutional racism. This may allow governments and institutions to deny or evade responsibility for systemic racism. Organisations who offer 'unconscious bias training' often claim that this shows that they have addressed racism, but this training can be used as a tactic to avoid having to address structural biases within the organisation. We have seen this in the case of the Metropolitan Police (Casey, 2023).

Ethnic Diversity in the UK

Archaeological evidence suggests that the earliest settlers in Britain in the Mesolithic era were hunter–gatherers, and DNA evidence shows that they were dark skinned. Farming practices then spread to Britain during the Neolithic era around 6000 years ago and are thought to have been brought here by migrants from modern-day Turkey. At this time, the skin colour of the population was extremely variable. A paler-skinned population only arrived later during further large-scale migrations to the UK from Northern Europe around 3000 years ago during the Bronze Age (Davies, 2019).

The population of the UK has thus been created from successive waves of mass migration over several millennia. In the first millennium AD, there were mass migrations by the Romans, Angles, Saxons, Vikings and, finally, the Normans during their Conquest of Britain in 1066 (Ashworth, 2022). As Britain became a global trading nation, and then an imperial power from the sixteenth century onwards, more waves of migration occurred. The Chinese and Lascar seamen from Asia settled in UK ports from the seventeenth century onwards. French Huguenot refugees arrived in the sixteenth and seventeenth centuries and Jewish refugees from Europe in the nineteenth and twentieth centuries. In the nineteenth century, people were also brought to the UK to work as a result of the industrial revolution. Many Irish people came to work in Britain at this time, especially after the Irish potato famine (Shankley et al., 2020).

Migration after World War II has also played a decisive role in shaping the ethnic make-up of the UK today. After the war, migration to the UK from Commonwealth countries was actively encouraged to rebuild the country. The newly created NHS recruited many staff from the

Commonwealth and, in particular, recruited nurses in the Caribbean (Baxter, 1988). This need for workers in the 1950s and 1960s also brought in significant numbers of South Asian migrants to work in manufacturing and service industries, particularly in the north of England (Shankley et al., 2020).

The ethnic make-up of the UK today is a result of all these successive waves of migration, with post-war migration playing a very important part. According to the 2021 census figures for England and Wales,

- 81.7% of the population describe themselves as 'White'. Seventy-five percent of this group describe themselves as British, English, Welsh, Northern Irish or Scottish. The remainder identify themselves in 'other' White categories, such as Irish.
- 9.3% of the population identify themselves as Asian British.
- 4% of the population identify themselves as Black British, Caribbean or African.
- 2.9% of the population Identify themselves as coming from a mixed heritage.
- 2.1% of the population identify themselves as belonging to 'other' ethnic groups (Office for National Statistics, 2022).

Thus, the UK, whilst having a predominantly White British population, has always been ethnically diverse and has become more ethnically diverse in the decades since World War II. Much of this diversity has occurred as a result of the post-war migration invited by UK governments to meet the country's economic needs. We can see this most clearly in the recruitment of NHS and social care staff from overseas, often to unpopular and under-resourced specialities (Tuffour, 2022).

Ethnic Inequality in the UK

There is considerable variation in the social circumstances of ethnic minority groups in the UK, but the key message is that, despite these variations, people from ethnic minority groups are more likely than the White population to be economically disadvantaged. Indian and Chinese people are to some extent an exception, doing better in work and education than other ethnic minority groups. Overall, however, there have been persistent ethnic inequalities in the job market in the UK, with people from ethnic minority backgrounds being more likely to be in low-paid and precarious work and twice as likely to be unemployed (Raleigh & Holmes, 2021). This cannot be explained by a lack of qualifications, since most ethnic minority groups had higher attainment at GCSE than the White British group in 2019–2020. Exceptions to this were Gypsy and Irish Travellers and males Black Caribbean pupils whose attainment was lower than other ethnic minority groups (Raleigh & Holmes, 2021). Ethnic minority students also have a higher rate of uptake of further and higher education, although they face more difficulties obtaining admission to elite universities (Shankley, 2020).

Inequality in the labour market is largely due to discrimination and stereotyping with people from ethnic minorities still not facing a level playing field when looking for work. This is shown by the fact that people from ethnic minority backgrounds are more likely to be overqualified for the job they are doing. Studies have also shown that they have to make more applications before being invited to job interviews if their ethnicity can be inferred from the information on their application form (Wilson, 2020).

ETHNIC MINORITIES AND POVERTY

As a result of these inequalities in the workplace, poverty is much higher among ethnic minorities with 53% of people of Bangladeshi origin and 48% of people of Pakistani origin living in poverty. The overall poverty rate for people of Black African, Black Caribbean and Black British heritage is around 40%. In comparison, White British people have a poverty rate of 20%, that is, half that of these ethnic minority groups (Joseph Rowntree Foundation, 2022). People from ethnic minority backgrounds are also more than twice as likely as White British people to be living in 'deep' poverty. 'Deep' poverty is defined as being more than 50% below the poverty line and creates difficult situations, such as people being forced to skip meals and choose between eating or heating their homes (Edmiston et al., 2022).

People from the poorest social classes are more likely to find themselves living in **deprived neighbourhoods** or what Marmot (2020) called the **'ignored places'** (see Chapter 2). However, people from ethnic minorities are at a higher risk of being forced into these areas than their White counterparts. Deprived neighbourhoods are measured on the basis of deficiencies in seven key factors:

- Low incomes
- Poor employment opportunities
- Poor access to health services
- Poor access to education services
- High crime levels
- Barriers to housing and other services, such as leisure and retail
- A poor living environment.

A **poor living environment** is described as a neighbourhood where a high proportion of housing is in poor condition and there is poor air quality alongside heavy traffic and high rates of road traffic accidents. Typically, there is also a lack of access to green spaces and an absence of street trees. Green spaces and street trees can play an important role in mitigating air pollution from traffic (Roe et al., 2016).

People from ethnic minorities are thus more likely to be exposed to a dangerous and health-damaging environment by being forced to live in this type of neighbourhood. In particular, they are more likely to be exposed to long-term air pollution. This, in turn, can lead to higher rates of long-standing illness (Al Ahad et al., 2022). Living in a deprived neighbourhood can compound problems of poverty and deprivation and make it harder to escape poverty due to poor employment opportunities, lack of access to services and the negative health effects of the environment (Salway et al., 2007). These areas also typically have much poorer access to health services due to the **'inverse care law'** (Marmot, 2018) (see Chapter 2). People from ethnic minorities are often pushed into these areas by a combination of poverty, discrimination and social exclusion (Almeida, 2021; Joseph Rowntree Foundation, 2013). Historic and contemporary institutional racism within the housing sector has played an important role in creating this situation. This was highlighted by the tragedy of the Grenfell Tower fire (Shankley & Finney, 2020).

Case Example: Poor Living Environments, Institutional Racism and Health

In 2022, a two-year-old toddler called Awaab Ishak died from a severe respiratory condition called granulomatous tracheobronchitis. At his inquest the coroner concluded that the illness that caused his death was due to exposure to mould in his housing association home in Rochdale. As his condition had worsened, his parents had repeatedly asked for the damp and mould to be addressed, as had the family's health visitor. During the time that Awaab was ill, the housing association made no effort to treat the mould or address the damp in his home. Instead, housing association officials had blamed the family's lifestyle and made racist assumptions including that the family engaged in 'ritual bathing' practices. They did not; they took showers just like everyone else. The coroner concluded that Awaab's life could have been saved if the housing association had acted.

(BARANUIK, 2023)

Baranuik (2023) suggests that people should be able to cook food and take a shower without these activities causing toxic problems in the home. However, he suggests that people living in unsafe housing are often blamed and 'gaslighted' (see Chapter 3) by their landlords, and this was the case for Awaab's family. This type of situation is disproportionately faced by people from ethnic minorities and can be seen as an example of institutional racism. In England, 3.5 million homes fail to meet the standard of a 'decent home' set by the UK government; over 2 million are sufficiently substandard to represent a serious threat to health and almost a million have a serious problem with damp and mould (Department for Levelling Up, Housing and Communities, 2020). People from ethnic minorities are more likely to experience housing disadvantage and to live in poor-quality, precarious and overcrowded housing. For example, 30% of Bangladeshi households are overcrowded compared to 2% of White households (Platt & Warwick, 2020). Ethnic minority people are also more likely to experience homelessness (Shankley & Finnay, 2020).

We have thus considered a number of different ways in which people from ethnic minorities can be subject to systemic disadvantages which can adversely impact on their health. To add insult to injury, there is evidence to suggest that people from ethnic minorities are often treated punitively and blamed for their predicament whether this involves living in poverty, poor housing or deprived neighbourhoods. Studies have uncovered both class prejudice and institutional racism within the state agencies that deal with the disadvantaged. This can lead to a punitive culture which **'others'** people suffering distress and disadvantage (Snoussi & Mompelat, 2019).

Othering describes the action of treating disenfranchised individuals or groups as essentially different and inferior to a dominant group. While the term has been used mainly to describe the racist othering of ethnic minority groups, it can also be applied to other disenfranchised groups including the poor, the old and people with disabilities. Othering involves categorising people as 'other' and 'not like us', invoking an 'us and them' mentality. Treating an individual as 'other' can be used to justify discrimination, poor treatment and denial of human rights. It is often based on distorted perceptions of minority groups as we saw in the case of Awaab Ishak above (Akbulut & Razum, 2022). In healthcare, it means not treating patients as individuals but instead as representatives of a category (Nye et al., 2023).

REFLECTION POINT

Review your understanding of the concept of institutional racism. To what extent do you think that the case of Awaab Ishak can be viewed as an example of institutional racism? How were Awaab and his family 'othered'? What could have been done to help Awaab and to prevent his avoidable death? What should be done in the future to prevent the deaths of children like Awaab?

Evidence of Ethnic Inequalities in Health

A growing body of evidence has indicated that people from some ethnic minority groups are more likely to have poor health than their White British counterparts. The picture is, however, complicated, as health inequalities linked to ethnicity intersect with other inequalities, such as class, gender and geographical area. There is also a lack of reliable, good-quality data on mortality rates. Ethnicity is not recorded when deaths are registered, so there are some big gaps in the data linking ethnicity to rates of death. As we do not have comprehensive mortality data, researchers instead have to try to link death records to other sources of data, such as hospital records, but this body of data also has gaps. The data on morbidity are more comprehensive and show that Bangladeshi, Pakistani, Gypsy and Irish Traveller groups have worse health across a range of different measures, followed by Caribbean and Indian people. White and Chinese people have the best health (Nazroo, 2003). The main measures of health showing these ethnic inequalities in overall health are self-reported health (Raleigh & Holmes, 2021) and disability-free life expectancy (Marmot, 2020; Wohland et al., 2015).

The recent COVID-19 pandemic disproportionately affected people from ethnic minorities who had both higher infection and mortality rates. This high COVID-19 mortality rate gave some ethnic minority groups a higher death rate than the White population, particularly during the first wave of the pandemic (Nazroo & Becares, 2021; Raleigh & Holmes, 2021). Many members of ethnic minorities were working in low-paid, key worker roles during the pandemic and thus at higher risk of exposure to infection. Ethnic minority healthcare staff also suffered higher rates of exposure to infection than their White colleagues (Kapadia et al., 2022). Social deprivation and the risks associated with living in substandard and overcrowded housing may also have played a part in the higher COVID-19 death rate among ethnic minorities (Morales & Ali, 2021).

Apart from a higher infection and mortality rate from COVID-19, ethnic minority groups have higher rates of illness and mortality from a number of specific conditions. In particular, the incidence prevalence and mortality from cardiovascular disease are higher among South Asians (people with Indian, Bangladeshi and Pakistani backgrounds). This is thought to be due to a mix of physiological susceptibility, social and environmental factors, such as poverty, and lifestyle factors, such as lack of exercise. Black groups (Black British, African and Caribbean) have a lower rate of heart disease but a higher prevalence of hypertension and higher incidence of stroke (Raleigh & Holmes, 2021).

The risk of developing diabetes is six times higher in South Asian groups than their White counterparts, and in Black groups it is three times higher. Again, a mix of physiological susceptibility, socioeconomic deprivation and lifestyle factors such as diet and exercise are thought to be responsible. Nazroo (2003), however, suggests that health inequalities linked to ethnicity are closely tied to socioeconomic position and that this is the most important factor explaining these inequalities. For example, a lifestyle factor cited as being linked to cardiovascular disease in South Asian populations is lack of exercise. Although culture is often cited as one reason for this, deprivation and discrimination are important factors. Living in a deprived neighbourhood with a lack of safe outside spaces and encountering racism in public spaces can deter people from participating in outdoor exercise.

Overall rates of cancer are lower among ethnic minority groups. This may be in part due to lower rates of smoking and alcohol consumption. However, this headline figure conceals higher rates of specific cancers in certain groups, such as a higher rate of liver and mouth cancer among South Asians and a higher rate of prostate cancer in Black British, Caribbean and African men. Lung cancer mortality is also higher among Bangladeshi men (Raleigh & Holmes, 2021).

There are also some marked inequalities in mental health. In general, people from ethnic minorities are more likely to have difficulty getting a diagnosis and treatment for a mental health problem. However, young Black Caribbean men are roughly six times more likely to be admitted to a psychiatric hospital with a serious mental illness, such as schizophrenia. The reasons for these disparities are hotly debated, and some authors see this as an example of 'Eurocentric' models of mental health care which are insensitive to the lived experiences and cultures of ethnic minority patients (Bansal et al., 2022).

There are stark differences in rates of maternal and infant mortality between ethnic minorities and the White population. The rate of deaths during pregnancy and childbirth amongst women from Black British, Caribbean and African backgrounds is four times that of White women. The rates of maternal mortality for Asian women are double those of White women. A House of Commons report highlighted three key factors. Firstly, women in these groups had a higher rate of pre-existing conditions, especially diabetes and hypertension. Secondly, ethnic minority women are more likely to be living in poverty and in deprived neighbourhoods. Finally, there is evidence that some ethnic minority women receive poorer standards of care, and we will consider this in more detail later in the chapter (Women and Equalities Committee, 2023). Infant mortality rates have also remained higher in ethnic minority groups due to the same factors (Raleigh & Holmes, 2021).

There are also marked ethnic inequalities in health in later life. Rates of poor self-rated health tend to increase in all ethnic groups after the age of 40, but this is particularly true of people from Pakistani and Bangladeshi backgrounds as well as for Black Caribbean men. For example, 22% of White women in their 80s report that their health is poor. A similar number of Pakistani women (23%) report the same level of poor health when they are only in their 50s (Centre for Ageing Better, 2021). Rates of multimorbidity are also higher amongst older people from ethnic minority groups (Hayanga et al., 2024). Socioeconomic deprivation plays an important part in these differences with the effects of deprivation accumulating across the life course.

We have thus seen that although there are still some gaps in our knowledge, there is a considerable amount of evidence showing a link between ethnicity and poor health. In the next section we will consider the explanations for ethnic inequalities in health in a little more detail.

EXPLANATIONS FOR ETHNIC INEQUALITIES IN HEALTH

Below we assess the four leading explanations that have been suggested to explain ethnic inequalities in health.

Biological Susceptibility

Explanations in terms of **biology** make assumptions about physiological differences between people from different ethnic backgrounds. As discussed earlier, in general, there is more biological variation within groups than between them. However, physiological differences exist to a limited degree in relation to specific conditions. Thus, susceptibility to haemoglobinopathies is linked to ethnic origins. For example, sickle cell disease is linked to West African, Middle Eastern, Caribbean and Indian ancestry while thalassemia is more prevalent in people with South East Asian, Mediterranean and Chinese ancestry. The role of physiology (as opposed to socioeconomic factors and lifestyle) in the susceptibility of South Asians to diabetes is still debated but there are some indications that insulin resistance is higher in the South Asian population making them more at risk of developing diabetes (Shah & Kanaya, 2014). It is likely that social factors (particularly poverty and deprivation) then compound this risk.

Culture and Lifestyle

A popular explanation suggests that ethnic inequalities in health are due to differences in **culture and behaviours**. This is often referred to as **'lifestyle factors'** and it is an attractive explanation for governments, policymakers and clinicians. Health inequalities are blamed on the very individuals suffering from these disadvantages and it is them that are asked to change their behaviour while their disadvantaged circumstances are ignored. This has the appeal of seeming to be a cheaper and easier fix for the problem of ethnic inequalities. Clinicians may also turn to behavioural explanations because they have no power to address structural disadvantages, such as poverty, so that lifestyle advice is the only thing that they have to offer. However, a lack of understanding of the structural causes of ethnic inequalities can have a negative impact when it leads clinicians to give judgmental care or give advice that patients simply don't have the means to follow. Williams suggests that:

> *'There is a temptation to focus on identified risk factors as the focal point for intervention efforts. In contrast, we indicate that the macro-social factors and racism are the basic causes of racial differences in health'.*

> (WILLIAMS ET AL., 1994, p. 36)

One of the problems about this focus on culture is firstly that it can often lead to crude (and sometimes racist) forms of blame and 'othering' as we saw in the case of Awaab Ishak. It also tends to operate with a deficit model focusing on problems rather than positive aspects of ethnic minority behaviours. For example, people from Pakistani and Bangladeshi backgrounds are rarely applauded for their lower rates of smoking and alcohol consumption. Secondly, crude assumptions about culture in respect of lifestyle factors, such as diet and exercise, also ignore the important impact of 'macro-social' and economic inequalities in shaping people's health. Cultural and behavioural explanations that ignore these structural factors can thus operate as a form of **victim blaming** (see Chapter 1).

Socioeconomic Deprivation

A third explanation focuses on the ways in which ethnic identity intersects with social class. As discussed earlier, there is a very strong case to be made for the importance of **inequalities in socioeconomic status** as a fundamental cause of ethnic inequalities of health. According to Link and Phelan (1995):

> *'A fundamental social cause involves resources that determine the extent to which people are able to avoid risks for morbidity and mortality' (p. 88).*

Thus, Phelan and Link (2015) identify a number of ways in which deprivation and poverty deprive people from ethnic minorities of the resources needed to keep themselves safe and healthy. They pay particular attention to the neighbourhood effects discussed earlier in this chapter. These include exposure to unwanted risks, such as environmental toxins, crime, drugs and traffic accidents as well as diminished access to the things that keep people healthy, such as safe spaces for recreation, affordable healthy food and good medical services. Thus socioeconomic deprivation directly exposes people to health hazards. It also harms health indirectly by limiting people's ability to engage in health-promoting behaviours, such as exercising and eating a healthy diet.

Nazroo (2003) also emphasises that research studies that take account of socioeconomic status show that ethnic inequalities are largely related to economic differentials. There is, however, some additional disadvantage for people from ethnic minorities not fully explained by socioeconomic status. This can largely be explained by the experience of racism.

The Experience of Racism

A fourth explanation is therefore that the **experience of racism and discrimination** has health-damaging effects which are cumulative. We talked earlier about exposures to **'micro aggressions'** (Golash-Boza, 2016). These experiences act as social stressors. Social stressors can cause physiological responses to threatening experiences that can damage health over time. The cumulative toll of the social stress caused by being the victim of racist acts leads over time to what has been described as a **'weathering'** effect. The concept of 'weathering' suggests that the stress of racism and stigmatisation causes cumulative wear and tear on the body's systems (Phelan & Link, 2015). Similarly, exposure to institutional racism can limit an individual's life chances as well as exposing them to stress.

It is likely that these stresses accumulate across the life course. Earlier we considered ethnic inequalities in health in later life and linked these to social deprivation. However, if we adjust the figures to take account of socioeconomic status, we can see that there is still an additional burden on health associated with being from Pakistani, Bangladeshi, Black Caribbean and Indian backgrounds when compared with people coming from a White British background. Studies have shown that this is correlated with self-reported exposure to racial discrimination so is likely to be due to the burden of dealing with racism across the life course (Centre for Ageing Better, 2021).

Inequity, Institutional Racism and Discrimination in Health and Care Services

We have discussed inequalities in the health status of people from ethnic minority backgrounds. In this section we will discuss **inequity** in health services. Inequity is closely related to inequality but is a slightly different concept. We use the term **inequity** to refer to avoidable differences in the provision of services to different groups. This also suggests a level of unfairness in both access to services and the quality of services received (Global Health Europe, 2009). Inequity in service provision can deepen inequalities between ethnic groups.

In this section we will consider whether inequity in the provision and delivery of health services contributes to ethnic inequalities in health. We talked earlier about institutional racism and here we will consider whether there are structural inequities in timely and appropriate access to services. We will also consider whether discrimination, racism, stereotyping or cultural incompetence affect the quality of care experienced by people from ethnic minorities. Two particular examples will be discussed here; maternity services and the impact of immigration policies on the provision of healthcare to ethnic minorities.

INSTITUTIONAL RACISM IN HEALTH AND CARE SERVICES

We talked earlier about institutional racism and we will now briefly examine evidence of institutional (or structural) racism in healthcare. Institutional racism in healthcare can occur whenever people from ethnic minority groups systematically receive suboptimal healthcare when compared to their White British counterparts. This can be due to institutional neglect of the particular needs of ethnic minority patients or a culture that tolerates or ignores discriminatory behaviour by staff, patients or visitors (Essex et al., 2022a). Neglect of the health of ethnic minority groups in medical and nursing education is another example of structural racism; for example, not teaching staff how to recognise cyanosis in a person with dark skin (Mukwende, 2020).

A failure to adequately meet the needs of ethnic minority patients can also result from resourcing decisions that mean that conditions mainly affecting ethnic minorities are systemically under-resourced as are services specifically for ethnic minority patients (Elias & Paradies, 2021). For example, screening for sickle cell disease and thalassemia was only introduced in 2003 and these services remain under-resourced (Chouhan & Nazroo, 2020). Similarly, interpreting services are patchy within the NHS and often poorly resourced and reliant on unpaid volunteers (Chouhan & Nazroo, 2020).

Health problems affecting ethnic minorities may also be under-researched. There has been a growing body of evidence, building since the 1980s, showing that pulse oximetry is less accurate in darker-skinned people and can underestimate their level of hypoxia. This poses risks for critically ill, ethnic minority patients (Kyriacou et al., 2023). This became particularly significant during the COVID-19 pandemic when the death rate amongst ethnic minority patients was high and there was heavy reliance on the pulse oximeter to triage patients and make treatment decisions (Crooks et al., 2022). It is concerning that this racial bias has been known for many years and yet still not addressed (NHS Race and Health Observatory, 2021).

Thus, structural racism can worsen care outcomes. It can also cause poor experiences of care. Studies have shown that ethnic minority patients report worse experiences of healthcare across a range of services. In primary care, studies have suggested that ethnic minority patients wait longer for appointments and are more dissatisfied with communication within the consultation (Chouhan & Nazroo, 2020). A finding of great concern is that ethnic minority patients with cancer have been shown to have needed to make more appointments with a GP than their White counterparts before being referred to a cancer specialist (Pinder et al., 2016). We will now consider two examples of inequity in care provision in a little more detail.

Maternal and Neonatal Care

We noted earlier that there were higher rates of maternal and infant mortality among mothers and babies from ethnic minority groups and that this appears to be, in part, due to poorer care. A Canadian study of South Asian women patients found that the participants experienced '**othering**' by healthcare staff (Johnson et al., 2004).

Othering practices that were found in (Johnson et al., 2004) study included negative overgeneralisations about South Asians which represented them as noncompliant, ignorant or coming from a 'backward' culture. A classic study of maternity care in the UK also found that midwives regarded Asian women as 'not the same as us'. Midwives in this study stereotyped Asian women as 'making a fuss' and saw Asian women as being 'all the same' but 'not like us'; thus both stereotyping and othering this group of patients (Bowler, 1993). Similarly, a recent study of birth notes in the United States found clinicians from a range of disciplines used stigmatising language in notes to describe ethnic minority mothers (Barcelona et al., 2023). It is unsurprising, therefore, that studies have reported that ethnic minority women receive fewer antenatal checks; less pain relief during labour; experience a higher rate of emergency caesareans and are less likely to report being treated with kindness or spoken to in a way they can understand (Henderson et al., 2013). It seems that 'othering' is a key contributing factor to suboptimal care.

A recent report has also shown that there are racial biases in some safety-critical aspects of maternity practice. The Apgar score, which is a standardised assessment of the health of a baby immediately after birth, contains an assessment of skin colour in which a healthy score is represented by a baby that is 'pink all over' (Adams & Grunebaum, 2014). It is clear that clinicians using this score are inadequately guided as to how to assess healthy skin colour in babies with darker skin. A review of neonatal assessment procedures by the NHS Race and Health Observatory (2023) found that procedures for assessing skin colour, cyanosis and jaundice could all disadvantage babies with darker skin leading to safety concerns. Thus, we can see that in maternity care there are problems of both racial bias by staff and institutionally racist biases in processes, procedures and measures which can lead to increased risks for ethnic minority mothers and babies.

Care of Migrants and the 'Hostile Environment' in Healthcare

In this last example, we will look at recent changes in the rights to healthcare of migrants and overseas visitors to the UK and consider how these have generally affected the care of ethnic minorities in the UK. In the aftermath of World War II, the United Nations Geneva Convention on Refugees defined a refugee as:

> '*someone who is unable or unwilling to return to their country of origin owing to a well-founded fear of being persecuted for reasons of race, religion, nationality, membership of a particular social group, or political opinion.*'

> (UNHCR, 2011)

The Convention also stated that refugees should not be returned to countries where they risked threats to their safety. In recent years, there has been increased movement across the globe as more people have found it necessary to flee war, persecution and famine. For example, in poor countries, people are being displaced by the impacts of climate change caused by excessive carbon emissions by people in rich countries. It seems likely that migration will increase in future decades as global warming renders parts of the world uninhabitable. The reaction of some rich countries, including the UK, has been to introduce increasingly restrictive immigration policies and to make it more difficult for migrants to reach a safe country and achieve refugee status. Members of the United Nations have agreed to a 'global compact' on refugees. They have agreed to attempt to address the root causes of migration by mitigating the factors that force people to flee their country of origin, as well as agreeing to provide safe migration routes for people fleeing persecution. However, many member states have failed to meet their commitments including the UK (UNHCR, 2018).

Refugees and asylum seekers often have significant health needs. Studies have shown that one in six asylum seekers have a physical health problem while two thirds have experienced stress-related anxiety and depression (Burnett & Peel, 2001). Those fleeing conflict zones are likely to have had the experience of trauma, such as torture or the violent death of a close relative (British Medical Association, 2019). Child migrants are particularly vulnerable to health problems (Harkensee & Andrew, 2021). However, migrants frequently experience barriers to using health services in the UK, even when eligible for care, as rules on access are confusing. Many are now fearful of using the NHS (Weller et al., 2019).

The NHS was set up to offer universal healthcare 'free at the point of use' to the population and until recently this included visitors to the UK as well as British citizens (including those who had lived outside the UK for a period of time). This is no longer the case. In the aftermath of the 2008 financial crisis, NHS charges were introduced for people not normally resident in the UK including British citizens living abroad. People arriving here on work or student visas were also charged an upfront fee as part of their visa application (McHale & Speakman, 2020). In 2012, the rules about charging migrants and overseas visitors hardened when the then Home Secretary, Teresa May, stated that she wished to introduce a 'really hostile environment for illegal immigrants' (Essex et al., 2022b). In 2017, an upfront charge of 150% of the cost of care was introduced for patients who could not prove that they were UK residents and treatment could be refused if they could not pay. People needing emergency care could be charged afterwards, or their debt transferred to private debt collectors.

The hostile environment policy also introduced mandatory data sharing between the NHS and the Home Office so that NHS data could be used for immigration purposes. A debt to the NHS can now be used as grounds for deportation (Essex et al., 2022a). Health professionals are now required to check patients' immigration status before treating them and so have been co-opted into the immigration control system (Griffiths & Yeo, 2021). McHale and Speakman (2020) have suggested that this undermines the 'covenant of trust' between patients and health professionals. Other authors have questioned the risks to public health and the scheme's cost-effectiveness, given the costly bureaucracy that it has imposed on the NHS (Shahvisi, 2019).

Case History: The 'Hostile Environment' and Healthcare

Simba Mujakachi moved to the UK with his family as a child when his father was granted asylum here after facing an arrest warrant in Zimbabwe for speaking out against the dictator, Robert Mugabe. When he left school, aged 18, Simba applied for asylum and was refused. Then, under the hostile environment policy, Simba started to be charged upfront for his treatment for a clotting disorder. Fearful that he would incur a debt to the NHS that could result in his deportation to Zimbabwe, Simba stopped attending his appointments and stopped receiving his medication. As a result of stopping his medication he suffered a stroke which left him in a coma for 2 weeks and permanently paralysed on one side. The NHS charged him £100,000 for his care. Eventually, after an

11-year battle, Simba won his appeal for refugee status and for his debt to the NHS to be revoked. Legal changes since this case mean that someone like Simba would now have fewer rights to claim refugee status.

(POLITIS, 2022)

In practice, the hostile environment policy has mainly affected two main groups of people: firstly, people caught up in the long delays in the processing of asylum claims; and secondly, people from ethnic minorities who have lived in the UK for a long time but cannot produce the required paperwork to prove their residence status. This was particularly true of members of the 'Windrush generation', especially those who had arrived as children. Some elderly members of the Windrush generation, who had lived, worked and paid taxes here for most of their lives, started to find themselves being charged for NHS care because the Home Office had lost the paperwork showing their right to be here; some were even deported. This was eventually rectified after a public outcry (McHale & Speakman, 2020). However, many members of ethnic minorities continue to find themselves interrogated about their right to care when accessing NHS services.

Snoussi and Mompelet (2019) have suggested that the increasing co-optation of health and welfare professionals into social control functions, such as immigration controls, is creating more punitive welfare cultures and a 'trust deficit' between ethnic minorities and health professionals. People from ethnic minority backgrounds can then feel dehumanised by bureaucracy when accessing services, while health professionals have acquired an unwanted new role as a 'street-level bureaucrat' (Lipsky, 2010). We will return to this issue in Chapter 9.

Health professionals working with ethnic minority patients need to have an understanding of the damaging effects of both individual and institutional racism on the health of ethnic minorities. We need to reflect on our attitudes and behaviours but, more importantly, be vigilant for signs of institutional racism in the organisations in which we work.

REFLECTION POINT

Think about a clinical setting in which you have worked. How well did it cater to the specific needs of ethnic minority patients that you encountered? Were there any ways in which you thought that the care of ethnic minorities could be institutionally racist? What changes would you recommend to the managers of this setting and why?

Summary of Key Points

- Historically, the UK has been an ethnically diverse country and has become more diverse since World War II.
- The UK has a history of colonialism that has left behind a legacy of institutionalised racism in some organisations.
- Many ethnic minorities suffer multiple disadvantages which include socioeconomic deprivation and the experience of racism and discrimination.
- Many ethnic minority groups suffer worse health than the White British population due to the multiple disadvantages that they suffer.
- There is some evidence of institutional racism with UK health services. This compromises standards of care.

Recommended Further Reading

Akala (2018). Natives: Race and class in the ruins of empire. Two Roads.

Byrne, B., Alexander, C., Khan, O., Nazroo, J., & Shankley, W. (2020). *Ethnicity, race and inequality in the UK: State of the Nation*. Policy Press.

Mukwende M. (2020). Mind the gap: A clinical handbook of signs and symptoms in black and brown skin. https://www.blackandbrownskin.co.uk/mindthegap

Sanghera, S. (2021). *Empireland: How imperialism has shaped modern Britain*. Penguin Books Ltd.

Snoussi, D., & Mompelat, L. (2019). *We are ghosts': Race, class and institutional prejudice*. Runnymede Trust.

References

Adams, B. N., & Grunebaum, A. (2014). Does "pink all over" accurately describe an Apgar color score of 2 in newborns of color? *Obstetrics & Gynecology, 123*, 36.

Akbulut, N., & Razum, O. (2022). Why Othering should be considered in research on health inequalities: Theoretical perspectives and research needs. *SSM-Population Health, 20*, 101286.

Al Ahad, M. A., Demšar, U., Sullivan, F., & Kulu, H. (2022). Does long-term air pollution exposure affect self-reported health and limiting long term illness disproportionately for ethnic minorities in the UK? A census-based individual level analysis. *Applied Spatial Analysis, 15*, 1557–1582.

Almeida, A. (2021). *Pushed to the margins: A quantitative analysis of gentrification in London in the 2010s*. Runnymede Trust.

Ashworth, J. (2022). *Early English Anglo-Saxons descended from mass European migration*. Natural History Museum. Retrieved December 11, 2023, from https://www.nhm.ac.uk/discover/news/2022/september/early-english-anglo-saxons-descended-from-mass-european-migration.html.

Bansal, N., Karlsen, S., Sashidharan, S. P., Cohen, R., Chew-Graham, C. A., & Malpass, A. (2022). Understanding ethnic inequalities in mental healthcare in the UK: A meta-ethnography. *PLoS Medicine, 19*, 12.

Baranuik, C. (2023). The doctor forcing landlords to act on mouldy homes. *BMJ, 380*, 698.

Barcelona, V., Scharp, D., Idnay, B. R., Moen, H., Goffman, D., Cato, K., & Topaz, M. (2023). A qualitative analysis of stigmatizing language in birth admission clinical notes. *Nursing Inquiry, 30*(3), e12557.

Baxter, C. (1988). *Black Nurse: An endangered species—A case for equal opportunities in nursing*. National Extension College Trust Ltd.

Bourne, J. (2019). Unravelling the concept of unconscious bias. *Race & Class, 60*(4), 70–75.

Bowler, I. (1993). 'They're not the same as us': Midwives' stereotypes of South Asian descent maternity patients. *Sociology of Health & Illness, 15*(2), 157–178.

British Medical Association. (2019). *BMA refugee and asylum seeker health resource*. Retrieved December 11, 2023, from https://www.bma.org.uk/media/1838/bma-refugee-and-asylum-seeker-health-resource-june-19.pdf.

Burnett, A., & Peel, M. (2001). Asylum seekers and refugees in Britain: Health needs of asylum seekers and refugees. *BMJ, 322*(7285), 544.

Cabinet Office. (2021). *Writing about Ethnicity*. Retrieved December 11, 2023, from https://www.ethnicity-facts-figures.service.gov.uk/style-guide/writing-about-ethnicity.

Casey, L. (2023). Baroness Casey review, final report, an independent review into the standards of behaviour and internal culture of the Metropolitan Police Service Metropolitan Police Service. Retrieved December 11, 2023, from https://www.met.police.uk/police-forces/metropolitan-police/areas/about-us/about-the-met/bcr/baroness-casey-review/.

Centre for Ageing Better. (2021). *Ethnic health inequalities in later life: The persistence of disadvantage from 1993–2017*. December 11, 2023, from https://ageing-better.org.uk/sites/default/files/2021-11/health-inequalities-in-later-life.pdf.

Chouhan, K., & Nazroo, J. (2020). Health inequalities. In B. Byrne, C. Alexander, O. Khan, J. Nazroo, & W. Shankley (Eds.), *Ethnicity, race and inequality in the UK: State of the Nation* (pp. 73–92). Policy Press.

Crooks, C. J., West, J., Morling, J. R., Simmonds, M., Juurlink, I., Briggs, S., & Fogarty, A. W. (2022). Pulse oximeter measurements vary across ethnic groups: An observational study in patients with COVID-19. *European Respiratory Journal, 59*(4), 1–4.

Davies, J. (2019). *Neolithic Britain: Where did the first farmers come from?* Natural History Museum. Retrieved December 11, 2023, from https://www.nhm.ac.uk/discover/news/2019/april/neolithic-britain-where-did-the-first-farmers-come-from.html.

Department for Levelling Up, Housing and Communities. (2020). *English housing survey housing: Quality and condition*. Retrieved December 11, 2023, from https://assets.publishing.service.gov.uk/government/uploads/system/uploads/attachment_data/file/1088447/EHS_Housing_quality_and_condition_report_2020.pdf.

Edmiston, D., Begum, S., & Kataria, M. (2022). *Falling faster amidst a cost-of-living crisis: Poverty, inequality and ethnicity in the UK*. Runnymede Trust.

Elias, A., & Paradies, Y. (2021). The costs of institutional racism and its ethical implications for healthcare. *Journal of Bioethical Inquiry, 18*, 45–58.

Essex, R., Markowski, M., & Miller, D. (2022a). Structural injustice and dismantling racism in health and healthcare. *Nursing Inquiry, 29*(1), e12441.

Essex, R., Riaz, A., Casalotti, S., Worthing, K., Issa, R., Skinner, J. S., & Yule, A. (2022b). A decade of the hostile environment and its impact on health. *Journal of the Royal Society of Medicine, 115*(3), 87–90.

Giddens, A., & Sutton, P. (2017). *Sociology*. Polity Press.

Global Health Europe (2009). Inequity and inequality in health. Retrieved December 11, 2023, from https://globalhealtheurope.org/values/inequity-and-inequality-in-health/.

Golash-Boza, T. (2016). A critical and comprehensive sociological theory of race and racism. *Sociology of Race and Ethnicity, 2*(2), 129–141.

Griffiths, M., & Yeo, C. (2021). The UK's hostile environment: Deputising immigration control. *Critical Social Policy, 41*(4), 521–544.

Harkensee, C., & Andrew, R. (2021). Health needs of accompanied refugee and asylum-seeking children in a UK specialist clinic. *Acta Paediatrica, 110*(8), 2396–2404.

Hayanga, B., Stafford, M., Saunders, C. L., & Bécares, L. (2024). Ethnic inequalities in age-related patterns of multiple long-term conditions in England: Analysis of primary care and nationally representative survey data. *Sociology of Health & Illness, 46*(4), 582–607.

Henderson, J., Gao, H., & Redshaw, M. (2013). Experiencing maternity care: The care received and perceptions of women from different ethnic groups. *BMC Pregnancy and Childbirth, 13*(1), 1–14.

Johnson, J. L., Bottorff, J. L., Browne, A. J., Grewal, S., Hilton, B. A., & Clarke, H. (2004). Othering and being othered in the context of health care services. *Health communication, 16*(2), 255–271.

Joseph Rowntree Foundation. (2013). *Ethnicity and deprivation in England: How likely are ethnic minorities to live in deprived neighbourhoods?* Retrieved December 11, 2023, from https://hummedia.manchester.ac.uk/institutes/code/briefingsupdated/ethnicity-and-deprivation-in-england-how-likely-are-ethnic-minorities-to-live-in-deprived-neighbourhoods%20(1).pdf.

Joseph Rowntree Foundation. (2022). *UK Poverty 2023: The essential guide to understanding poverty in the UK*. Retrieved December 11, 2023, from https://www.jrf.org.uk/report/uk-poverty-2023.

Kapadia D., Zhang J., Salway S., Nazroo J., Booth A., Villarroel-Williams N., Bécares L., Esmail A. (2022). Ethnic Inequalities in HealthCare: A rapid evidence review. Retrieved December 11, 2023, from https://www.nhsrho.org/research/ethnic-inequalities-in-healthcare-a-rapid-evidence-review-2/.

Kyriacou, P. A., Charlton, P. H., Al-Halawani, R., & Shelley, K. H. (2023). Inaccuracy of pulse oximetry with dark skin pigmentation: Clinical implications and need for improvement. *British Journal of Anaesthesia, 130*(1), e33–e36.

Link, B. G., & Phelan, J. C. (1995). Social conditions as fundamental causes of disease. *Journal of Health and Social Behavior, 35*(Extra issue), 80–94.

Lipsky, M. (2010). *Street-level bureaucracy: Dilemmas of the individual in public services*. Russell Sage Foundation.

Macpherson, L. (1999). *The Stephen Lawrence Inquiry, Cm. 4262–I*. Stationary Office.

Marmot, M. (2018). An inverse care law for our time. *BMJ, 31*, 362.

Marmot, M. (2020). Health equity in England: The Marmot review 10 years on. *BMJ, 368*, m693.

McHale, J. V., & Speakman, E. M. (2020). Charging 'overseas visitors' for NHS treatment, from Bevan to Windrush and beyond. *Legal Studies, 40*(4), 565–588.

Morales, D. R., & Ali, S. N. (2021). COVID-19 and disparities affecting ethnic minorities. *The Lancet, 397*(10286), 1684–1685.

Mukwende, M. (2020). *Mind the gap: A clinical handbook of signs and symptoms in black and brown skin*. Retrieved December 11, 2023, from https://www.blackandbrownskin.co.uk/mindthegap.

Nazroo, J., & Becares, L. (2021). *Ethnic inequalities in COVID-19 mortality: A consequence of persistent racism*. Runnymede Trust. Retrieved December 11, 2023, from https://www.runnymedetrust.org/publications/ethnic-inequalities-in-covid-19-mortality-a-consequence-of-persistent-racism.

Nazroo, J. (2003). The structuring of ethnic inequalities in health: economic position, racial discrimination, and racism. *American Journal of Public Health, 93*(2), 277–284.

NHS Race and Health Observatory (2021). Pulse oximetry and racial bias: Recommendations for national healthcare, regulatory and research bodies. Retrieved December 11, 2023, from https://www.nhsrho.org/

research/pulse-oximetry-and-racial-bias-recommendations-for-national-healthcare-regulatory-and-research-bodies/.

NHS Race and Health Observatory (2023). Review of neonatal assessment and practice in black, Asian, and minority ethnic newborns: Executive summary. Retrieved December 11, 2023, from file:///C:/Users/Hannah/Documents/Book2023/raceandethnicity/RHO-Neonatal_Executive-Summary.pdf.

Nye, C. M., Canales, M. K., & Somayaji, D. (2023). Exposing othering in nursing education praxis. *Nursing Inquiry, 30*(3), e12539.

Office for National Statistics (ONS). (2022). *Statistical bulletin, Ethnic group, England and Wales: Census 2021*. Retrieved December 11, 2023, from https://www.ons.gov.uk/peoplepopulationandcommunity/culturalidentity/ethnicity/bulletins/ethnicgroupenglandandwales/census2021.

Phelan, J. C., & Link, B. G. (2015). Is racism a fundamental cause of inequalities in health? *Annual Review of Sociology, 41*, 311–330.

Pinder, R. J., Ferguson, J., & Møller, H. (2016). Minority ethnicity patient satisfaction and experience: Results of the National Cancer Patient Experience Survey in England. *BMJ Open, 6*(6), e011938.

Platt, L., & Warwick, R. (2020). *Are some ethnic groups more vulnerable to Covid-19 than others?* The Institute for Fiscal Studies. Retrieved December 11, 2023, from https://www.ifs.org.uk/inequality/wp-content/uploads/2020/04/Are-some-ethnic-groups-more-vulnerable-to-COVID-19-than-others-V2-IFS-Briefing-Note.pdf.

Politis, M. (2022). Patient's £100 000 NHS debt is revoked as he is granted refugee status after 11 year battle. *BMJ, 377*, o1503.

Raleigh, V., & Holmes, J. (2021). *The health of people from ethnic minority groups in England*. King's Fund. Retrieved December 11, 2023, from https://www.kingsfund.org.uk/publications/health-people-ethnic-minority-groups-england.

Roe, J., Aspinall, P. A., & Ward Thompson, C. (2016). Understanding relationships between health, ethnicity, place and the role of urban green space in deprived urban communities. *International Journal of Environmental Research and Public Health, 13*(7), 681.

Said, E. W. (1978). *Orientalism*. Routledge Kegan Paul.

Salway, S., Platt, L., Chowbey, P., Harriss, K., & Bayliss, E. (2007). *Long-term ill health, poverty and ethnicity*. Joseph Rowntree Foundation, The Policy Press.

Sanghera, S. (2021). *Empireland: How imperialism has shaped Modern Britain*. Penguin Books Ltd.

Shah, A., & Kanaya, A. M. (2014). Diabetes and associated complications in the South Asian population. *Current Cardiology Rreports, 16*, 1–16.

Shahvisi, A. (2019). Austerity or xenophobia? The causes and costs of the "hostile environment" in the NHS. *Health Care Analysis, 27*(3), 202–219.

Shankley, W., & Rhodes, J. (2020). 'Racisms in contemporary Britain'. In B. Byrne, C. Alexander, O. Khan, J. Nazroo, & W., Shankley (Eds.), *Ethnicity, race and inequality in the UK: State of the Nation* (pp. 203–228). Policy Press.

Shankley, W. (2020). 'Ethnic inequalities in the state education system in England'. In B. Byrne, C. Alexander, O. Khan, J. Nazroo, & W. Shankley (Eds.), *Ethnicity, race and inequality in the UK: State of the Nation* (pp. 93–126). Policy Press.

Shankley, W., & Finney, N. (2020). Ethnic Minorities and Housing in Britain. In B. Byrne, C. Alexander, O, Khan. J. Nazroo, & W. Shankley (Eds.), *Ethnicity, race and inequality in the UK: State of the Nation* (pp. 149–166). Policy Press.

Shankley, W., Hannemann, T., & Simpson, L. (2020). The demography of ethnic minorities in Britain. In B. Byrne, C. Alexander, O. Khan, J. Nazroo, & W. Shankley (Eds.), *Ethnicity, race and inequality in the UK: State of the Nation* (pp. 15–34). Policy Press.

Snoussi, D., & Mompelat, L. (2019). *We are ghosts': Race, class and institutional prejudice*. Runnymede Trust.

Solomos, J. (2003). *Race and Racism in Britain*. Palgrave Macmillan.

Storm, I., Sobolewska, M., & Ford, R. (2017). Is ethnic prejudice declining in Britain? Change in social distance attitudes among ethnic majority and minority Britons. *The British Journal of Sociology, 68*(3), 410–434.

Tuffour, I. (2022). It is like 'judging a book by its cover': An exploration of the lived experiences of Black African mental health nurses in England. *Nursing Inquiry, 29*(1), e12436.

UN High Commissioner for Refugees (UNHCR). (2011). *The 1951 convention relating to the status of refugees and its 1967 protocol*. Retrieved December 11, 2023, from https://www.refworld.org/docid/4ec4a7f02.html.

UNESCO. (1978). Declaration on race and racial prejudice. Retrieved December 11, 2023, from https://en.unesco.org/about-us/legal-affairs/declaration-race-and-racial-prejudice.

UNHCR. (2018). *Global compact on refugees*. https://www.refworld.org/docid/63b43eaa4.html.

Weller, S. J., Crosby, L. J., & Turnbull, E. R. (2019). The negative health effects of hostile environment policies on migrants: A cross-sectional service evaluation of humanitarian healthcare provision in the UK. *Wellcome Open Research, 4*, 109.

Williams, D. R., Lavizzo-Mourey, R., & Warren, R. C. (1994). The concept of race and health status in America. *Public Health Reports, 109*(1), 26.

Wilson, T. (2020). *Racial inequality in the labour market has persisted for decades—We all have to play a part in addressing it*. Institute of Employment Studies. Retrieved December 11, 2023, from https://www.employment-studies.co.uk/news/racial-inequality-labour-market-has-persisted-decades-%E2%80%93-we-all-have-play-part-addressing-it.

Wohland, P., Rees, P., Nazroo, J., & Jagger, C. (2015). Inequalities in healthy life expectancy between ethnic groups in England and Wales in 2001. *Ethnicity & Health, 20*(4), 341–353.

Women and Equalities Committee. (2023). Black maternal health: Third report of session 2022–2023. House of Commons. Retrieved December 11, 2023, from https://committees.parliament.uk/publications/38989/documents/191706/default/.

PART 2

Health and Illness as Social and Cultural Experiences

Culture, Identity and the Body

Understanding Bodies

Health professionals are used to seeing the body in purely biological terms. We learn about its structure (anatomy) and functions (physiology) and how these can be changed by illness. However, our biology is only partly responsible for how we experience our bodies. We can also think of bodies as **'socially constructed'** (see Chapter 3) in that our perceptions and feelings towards our bodies, and the ways in which we use our bodies, are shaped by society and culture from an early age. These can, in turn, shape and change the physical properties of our bodies. For example, in a culture where women are expected to be submissive, women may learn to adopt a submissive posture in which the head is bowed. This can lead not only to permanent physical changes in the spine but also to a different view of the world; of the ground beneath women's feet rather than the view ahead. By contrast, the 'manly' man is expected to stand up straight with a direct and confident gaze upon the world around him (Bourdieu, 2013).

In this chapter we will consider how culture affects our perceptions and beliefs about our bodies. We discussed the concept of culture in Chapter 1. To recap briefly, when we talk about culture we are referring to the 'way of life' of a particular society including its language, customs, values, beliefs, social behaviours and rituals. We will also consider how our knowledge about our bodies is shaped by our social environment. Society and culture shape not only what we think about our bodies but also how we feel about our bodies. Culture affects whether we feel comfortable 'in our skin' and accept our bodies, or are dissatisfied, embarrassed or unhappy about them. These feelings about our bodies are influenced by the cultural ideas about the body which are prevalent in a society in a particular era.

Culture also affects how we care for our bodies and how we use and treat them in everyday activities. It can affect our posture and how we move about as well as our daily habits of body maintenance, such as eating, drinking, washing, dressing etc. More obviously, culture influences whether we decide to engage in projects to modify our bodies in response to cultural ideals. These **'body projects'** can range from diet and exercise programmes to tattooing, piercing, cosmetic surgery, dental reconstruction and 'gender-affirming' surgery. In an ageist society, there is also pressure to engage in body projects that hide the signs of ageing. At its most extreme, the preoccupation with reconstructing one's own body to conform to a desired or idealised body image can lead to illnesses, such as anorexia (see Chapter 3). One reason for the increased interest in the 'sociology of the body' is the enormous growth in these 'body projects' and the commercial industries associated with them. It has been suggested that in contemporary society we have been increasingly encouraged to objectify our own bodies, to see them as separate from ourselves and as something that should be worked on and changed rather than accepted. This attitude to our bodies would have seemed quite alien in some previous eras.

As health professionals, we engage in 'body work'. We handle, treat and manipulate other people's bodies. Nurses, in particular, frequently carry out body maintenance activities that an individual would normally carry out themselves, such as feeding, washing and adjusting bodily posture. Our work thus violates cultural norms (Lawler, 2006). We invade a person's personal space. We inspect parts of the body they would normally expect to keep private. We assist with highly personal body care practices, such as toileting. These encounters can be threatening to both parties. To successfully manage these encounters without evoking embarrassment or shame involves sensitive social judgements. These can be aided by a good understanding of the influence of society and culture on how both health professionals and patients understand and experience their bodies (Twigg, 2011). It is, therefore, important for health professionals to be knowledgeable about how people understand their bodies.

BODY KNOWLEDGE

We will start this chapter with a very simple question. What do people today know about their bodies? We live in an information-rich world with multiple TV channels, print media and the internet providing news and opinions about health and body maintenance. In theory, at least, people should be better informed about their bodies than ever before. However, the reality is somewhat different. Social scientists have researched the public's understanding of their bodies and found a complex picture in which medical knowledge is mixed with experiential knowledge as well as cultural beliefs and ideas.

Early studies of the public's understandings of the body investigated the levels of what was then paternalistically described as 'medical ignorance' among the general public. A study by Boyle in 1970 asked hospital outpatients to locate eight major organs on a picture of a human body. He found that the locations of organs were correctly identified only 50% of the time. A more recent study of the anatomical knowledge of hospital patients found that patients' knowledge had not improved much following the advent of the internet (Weinman, 2009). Even people with specific organ disease, such as kidney failure, were often uncertain about where the organs in question were located. Overall, patients had a less than 50% chance of correctly locating the position and size of organs, such as the lungs, ovaries, stomach, kidneys and heart (Weinman, 2009).

Thus, a substantial number of members of the public have only a hazy understanding of anatomy, that is, how their bodies are structured. When we consider how the public understand how their body functions, that is, its physiology, we find a similar story in which scientific knowledge is mixed with what have been called 'lay' beliefs. People form an understanding of their body which is shaped by two key factors: **culture** and **personal experience.** Scientific knowledge may form some part of an individual's understanding of their body but this is mixed in with personal experience and cultural ideas. Even people with in-depth medical knowledge, such as doctors, will be influenced by the cultural understandings of the body which they learnt growing up. Cultural understandings of the body have some deep roots as we will consider next.

HUMORAL MEDICINE

Modern biomedical ideas began to develop in Europe from the eighteenth century. Prior to this, medical practice in European societies had been dominated for 2000 years by humoral medicine.

BLOOD	YELLOW BILE
Personality: Sanguine	Personality: Melancholic
Properties: Hot and wet	Properties: Hot and dry
Element: Air	Element: Fire
PHLEGM	BLACK BILE
Personality: Phlegmatic	Personality: Choleric
Properties: Cold and wet	Properties: Cold and dry
Element: water	Element: earth

Fig. 5.1   The humoral system.

These ideas were first recorded by the Greek physician Hippocrates (460–370BC). In Hippocratic theory, the body contained four bodily fluids known as humours. These four humours corresponded to four elements that Greek philosophers believed made up all matter. These were earth, water, fire and air. The four humours believed to make up the body were blood, yellow bile, phlegm and black bile. Doctors practicing humoral medicine believed that illness was caused by an imbalance of these four humours and health could be restored by restoring balance. Thus, a deficiency in one of the humours might be addressed by altering the patient's diet or environment while an excess was dealt with by practices, such as the use of leeches, bleeding, starvation and cupping. Personality types and disorders were also linked to an imbalance in the humours; an excess of blood was believed to produce a sanguine (optimistic) temperament; black bile, a choleric (bad tempered) personality; phlegm, a phlegmatic (cool and unemotional) personality and yellow bile, a melancholic (despondent) personality (Porter, 2003). These ideas are summarised in Fig. 5.1.

Similar beliefs exist in other cultures and the idea that medicine was concerned with correcting an imbalance of the basic elements that constituted the body took different forms in different cultures. In the Indian Ayurvedic system of medicine, the body is believed to have three fundamental humours called vata, pitta and kapha which must be kept in balance. Similarly, in Chinese medicine, health is related to the harmonious balance of yin and yang. It is important to remember that these medical ideas linked traditional medicine to a wider set of religious and spiritual beliefs about the universe and our place in it which were fundamentally different to modern biomedicine. Today, these ideas underpin many alternative or complementary therapies, such as acupuncture. The idea of keeping elements of the body in some sort of balance has persisted in many popular health beliefs and practices.

The next question is just how far these ideas still influence people's beliefs' about how their body functions today. The medical anthropologist and doctor, Cecil Helman, suggested that the ideas of humoral medicine have left behind a legacy of folk beliefs about the body. He said that these folk beliefs help to explain how patients understand the inner workings of their bodies; how they believe their bodies are affected by external factors, such as diet and climate and what they believe about the body's by-products, such as urine, faeces and menstrual blood (Helman, 2007). Anthropology is a sister discipline to sociology which studies the development of human societies and it has a particular focus on culture.

In 1978, Helman published a study of his patients' beliefs about the causes of colds and flu. He found that patients commonly believed that colds or 'chills' were caused by getting cold or wet, whereas 'fevers', such as flu, were seen as 'hot' illnesses caused by 'germs', 'viruses' or 'bugs', though these terms were not used in the usual medical sense. He believed that although patients used some biomedical language, their understanding of the causes of illness had roots in humoral medicine. Thus, illnesses that caused 'phlegm' were linked to exposure to cold and wet just as in humoral medicine. Baer et al., (2008) found similar lay associations between getting cold and wet and catching the common cold in a cross-cultural study. They noted a hot–cold classification of illnesses across a variety of North American and South American cultures. Similarly, a number of studies of South Asians' beliefs about diabetes have noted the prevalence of a hot–cold system linked to the humoral ideas of Ayurvedic medicine (Greenhalgh et al., 1998).

Culture, Lived Experience and the Lifeworld

A more recent study by Prior et al., (2011) of how lay people talk about colds and flu also noted that while lay understanding intersected with biomedical knowledge it also contained many differences. Lay people put more emphasis on what was described as 'resistance' to illness which was believed to be associated with a variety of internal and external factors. Similar to Helman, Prior and others found many lay participants believed that resistance could be lowered by 'getting wet' or 'getting cold'. They also found that some participants believed that they had built up 'good resistance' over their lifetime and thus were 'resilient' people. Resistance was seen as similar to money in the bank saved up by a lifetime of 'good' habits. There were strong moral overtones to what were believed to constitute 'good' habits. Thus, lay ideas about 'good habits' mix medical prescriptions for a healthy lifestyle with moral judgements and folk beliefs handed down through generations. These beliefs were then cited as reasons why people refused a flu vaccination; they believed they had built up 'good resistance' through 'good habits' and that the 'flu jab' could threaten this.

Examples: Talking About Colds and Flu

> 'Well, I would catch it if I was out in the rain and I got soaked through. Then I would get the flu. I mean my neighbour up here was soaked through and he got pneumonia and he died. He was younger than me: well, 70. And he stayed in his wet clothes and that's fatal. Got pneumonia and died, but like I said, if I get wet, especially if I get my head wet, then I can get a nasty head cold and it could develop into flu later'.

> 'Because I'm fairly healthy. As a matter of fact … no, I don't want [the flu jab] now because I had shingles two years ago and I think I'm protected against the plague even.'

> (PRIOR ET AL., 2011, pp. 924–926)

Helman also suggested that lay people also draw symbolically on the world around them to make sense of how their body works. He said lay people often use metaphors to understand the workings of the body, such as the model that he called the 'plumbing model' of the body. In this model, internal organs are seen as a series of cavities connected by pipes. Problems are believed to occur when a pipe has become blocked. Helman says that this metaphorical thinking explains the popularity of expectorants and laxatives which in lay thinking give the body a 'good clear out' (Helman, 2007). A contemporary version of this might be the fashion for 'cleansing' and 'detoxification'. Increasingly, in contemporary society, people also liken the body to a machine in which parts can be fixed and replaced when they break or wear out (Poku et al., 2020). This latter metaphor may encourage people to objectify their bodies. Helman believed it could also give people unrealistic expectations of what modern medicine can fix.

Prior et al., (2011) suggest that lay people form beliefs about the workings of their body and its susceptibility to illness by drawing on a constellation of different sources. They suggest that they draw their understanding from dominant cultural ideas, personal experiences and what they call the 'small world' around them. Thus, they suggest, anecdotes about their own personal experiences and also the experiences of family, friends and neighbours loom large in lay people's accounts of how they make sense of their bodies, their health and their susceptibility to illness (Prior et al., 2011) (See also Chapter 6).

We can see therefore that people interpret and understand their bodies through their **lived experience** of their bodies but also through their experience of their immediate social world. The concepts of **embodiment** and of the **lifeworld** can help us to understand how people make sense of the world through their subjective experiences in everyday life. Both of these concepts originated in phenomenology.

Phenomenology is a branch of philosophy that is concerned with the nature of being. The discipline of phenomenology was founded by the German philosopher Edmund Husserl (1859–1938) and later developed further by the philosophers Martin Heidegger and Maurice Merleau-Ponty. Phenomenologists study human experience and consciousness. The American sociologist, Alfred Schutz, developed a phenomenological perspective within sociology. He saw the primary purpose of sociology as the study of human experience. Phenomenology underpins a style of qualitative research which is focused on understanding the lived experience of individuals. In healthcare, it is used primarily to understand patients' lived experiences of illness.

The term **embodiment** originated in the work of the French philosopher Maurice Merleau-Ponty (1908–1961). The term refers to the bodily elements of human subjectivity. We experience the social world through our bodies. For example, we may blush or feel overheated in awkward or embarrassing social situations. These physical sensations are manifestations of our emotions but can also act on our emotions and ultimately alter our outlook on the world. For example, we may learn to avoid social situations which make us feel physically uncomfortable. Phenomenology, therefore, distinguishes between the 'objective body', that is, the body as a physiological entity and the subjective body as uniquely experienced by each individual. Embodiment refers to the way in which our consciousness of the world is grounded in our bodily experience of it. People therefore experience and understand their bodies and bodily symptoms subjectively.

The term **lifeworld** originated in the work of Edmund Husserl to mean the world 'as lived'. In sociology, Schutz used the word pragmatically to mean our shared experience and understanding of the world. He was interested in how our relations with others affect our own subjective understanding of the world and he called these relations intersubjectivity (Ritzer, 2008). According to Schutz, people create their own social reality but do so in circumstances that are constrained by the social and cultural structures within which they live out their lives. Schutz called the everyday world in which people lived out their lives the **lifeworld.** In Schutz's work, the term **lifeworld** refers to people's everyday shared experiences as well as the commonsense assumptions that they employ to make sense of their experiences and the world around them (Ritzer, 2008).

More recently, sociologists, such as Pierre Bourdieu et al., (1999), have considered how social structures and particularly inequalities of wealth and power have shaped and influenced people's embodied experiences and lifeworld. We have seen this in the chapters on inequalities of class, gender and ethnicity.

We can conclude this section by saying that, although everyone has their own individual lifeworld shaped by their unique embodied experiences, they also live in an intersubjective world which is shaped by shared cultural understandings that have been handed down through generations. While individuals form their beliefs as a result of their own embodied experiences, these beliefs are also shaped through interaction with others, as well as the ideas they encounter in formal education and the media. These diverse ideas and experiences act as filters through which the biomedical model of the body is viewed. Lay people may therefore use medical terminology but understand it differently than health professionals. Similarly, while health professionals may understand and use the biomedical model, their judgements and attitudes may still be influenced by learned cultural beliefs about the body.

Culture and the Control of Bodily Functions

The concept of embodiment suggests that we experience the social world through our bodies while, at the same time, culture and society influence how we understand and experience our bodies. In this section we will be thinking about how we feel about our bodies and how we judge the bodies of other people. We will examine how cultural and social institutions shape and influence these feelings. We noted in the previous section how moral judgements entered into people's judgements about good and bad bodily habits. In this section we will consider these moral judgements further and examine two different theorists (Norbert Elias and Mary Douglas) who have suggested that they form part of a wider system of social order and control. Social disapproval can act as a powerful form of control over individuals and can provoke a range of negative emotions, such as shame, fear and disgust. We will look at how these systems of social disapproval and social control developed and their implications for people with particular body differences or problems.

CIVILISED BODIES

The sociologist Norbert Elias produced a major work called 'The Civilising Process' (Elias, 2012) which charted long-term processes of social development in Western Europe and the changes in manners and socially acceptable behaviour that accompanied them. Of particular interest to health professionals is his description of the way in which many bodily functions came to be seen as offensive and so came to be controlled or hidden. He asked the question: why are people in modern societies much more secretive about bodily functions, such as urinating and passing wind than people were in earlier times? His answer linked these changes in bodily habits to political and economic changes in European societies (Linklater & Mennell, 2010).

Elias suggested that the Middle Ages was a relatively lawless era in which violence was a fairly common and accepted way to settle personal disputes. By today's standards, behaviours and emotions were subject to far fewer restraints so, for example, there were fewer sanctions against fighting, urinating and spitting in public places. Elias then suggested that as the state grew, it imposed more control over citizens by acquiring a monopoly over legitimate violence. For example, it was no longer okay for ordinary people to settle their differences in public brawls as this threatened social order. Individual violence became much more strongly policed by the state and there was increasing pressure on individuals to exercise self-restraint in their emotions and behaviours.

Elias said that important reasons for this were that as society became more complex people became more interdependent and, in particular, strangers were more frequently forced into close proximity by urban living. This made self-restraint a desirable attribute. Elias researched these changes through looking at manuals on conduct and etiquette and the ways in which these changed through the centuries. Using these sources, Elias gives a forensic account of how new and stricter codes of polite behaviour came to govern a host of activities of daily living, such as eating, washing, dressing, urinating, defecating and nose-blowing. It was no longer okay to blow your nose on your sleeve or eat with your hands and using cutlery became obligatory (Elias, 2012).

In all these different areas, greater restraint was required and many bodily functions came to be seen as shameful acts that should be concealed or carried out in private (Nettleton, 2006). Identity, instead of being associated with family or clan, came to be more individualised and dependent on conformity to codes of social behaviour. Physical self-containment became a particularly important standard of conduct. Strong new rules were attached to the management of body fluids and odours. These rules occurred before there was an understanding of infection and germ theory which highlights the fact that they developed for social control reasons. Eventually, according to Elias, these standards of conduct were inculcated into infants from an early age (for example, through toilet training) so that they became part of an individual's **habitus**. The term *habitus* has been used in phenomenology by philosophers, such as Merleau-Ponty. In Elias's work, habitus refers to habits and dispositions that are so socially ingrained that they are no longer consciously thought about but seem to be 'second nature'. The term has gained particular currency in the sociological work of Pierre Bourdieu (see Chapter 2). When Bourdieu uses this term, he is also referring to the ways in which a person's habitus is structured by inequalities, such as social class and gender (Bourdieu, 2013).

While Elias saw the prohibitions surrounding bodily functions in modern society as linked to the 'civilising process', anthropologists, such as Mary Douglas have seen them as a much more enduring feature of human cultures. For example, taboos surrounding menstruation have a long history and have persisted across cultures (Gottlieb, 2020). According to Douglas, all societies have classification systems which identify what its culture defines as 'pure' or 'impure' (Douglas, 2003). Substances are considered polluting and subject to taboo if they are seen as violating a culture's systems of classification. Douglas sees human classification systems as essential to social cohesion and order. Thus, according to Douglas, what we consider dirty is anything which disrupts the normal order of things by breaching or blurring established boundaries. Dirt, she says, is simply 'matter out of place'. For example, spitting is viewed with strong social disapproval. When saliva is contained in the mouth it is considered 'clean' and thus we do not feel physical revulsion when kissing a loved one. However, when we spit it out, saliva is considered 'dirty' and then even our own saliva can stimulate a feeling of disgust. Douglas says these reactions are not based on hygiene theory but are deep-seated expressions of cultural norms. We will now consider how these cultural codes and taboos affect people who have difficulties controlling bodily fluids or odours.

'Leaky' Bodies

A study by Lawton (1998) of hospice care suggested more people now die at home and thus inpatient care is normally reserved for people with intractable symptoms. Prominent among these symptoms are conditions that cause leakage of body fluids, such as fungating wounds and faecal or urinary incontinence. She described these patients as having 'unbounded' bodies since in different ways they experienced the breakdown of the boundaries of their bodies. She then described the various social rejections that these individuals suffered and the deep sense of shame and degradation felt by the patients themselves. Their bodies felt 'out of control' and profoundly threatened their self-identity. Patients with 'unbounded' bodies often 'switched off' and became profoundly withdrawn in the last weeks of their lives. This loss of personhood is often described as '**social death**' and it occurs when people are socially rejected. Lawton suggests that the profound loss of personhood that these patients experienced is linked to the central importance that our culture places on self-control and the maintenance of what she calls a 'bounded, sealed, isolated body' (p. 138).

Case Example: Unbounded Bodies

Lawton describes the case of Annie; a woman in her 60s with a husband and son, who was admitted to the hospice for palliative care with cancer of the cervix. Her mobility had been affected by lymphoedema but the most prominent symptom which led to her admission was a recto-vaginal fistula which was causing faecal and urinary incontinence. Annie had wanted to stay at home until her death but she had herself requested admission to the hospice due to her feelings of shame and distress about her worsening incontinence. Her incontinence deteriorated further in the hospice causing intractable diarrhoea and bleeding. She also developed a urinary infection which both worsened the incontinence and caused a persistent unpleasant odour. She began to experience social rejection as other patients complained about the smell and asked to be moved. She was adamant that she did not want to be moved to a side ward so instead the patients around her gradually moved to other areas of the hospice. She became increasingly distressed and isolated and eventually requested sedation. She was then heavily sedated for the last two weeks of her life and nursed in a side ward. By the time of her death her family had ceased to visit and she died alone.

(LAWTON, 1998, pp. 124–127)

Lawton's study involved people at the end of life. However, some normal bodily functions, such as menstruation, can also create challenges for maintaining culturally expected bodily boundaries. Carter (2010) suggests that some pregnant women may experience the leakage of fluids, such as breast milk, as troubling and experience their bodies as 'out of control'. Pregnancy signifies new life, not death, yet the cultural demand to maintain physical self-control can also complicate women's experience of pregnancy. Lawton's study does not consider gender differences, but other authors have suggested that women are more likely to experience 'leaky' bodies (Jordan, 2007). The 'bounded, sealed, isolated body' described by Lawton may be a particularly masculine ideal.

Urinary incontinence is a common condition but one that sufferers find profoundly embarrassing. Peake and Manderson (2003) found that around a third of middle-aged women experienced episodes of incontinence regularly. Women in their study considered incontinence to be deeply shameful and coped by hiding it. This seriously restricted their lives and meant treatable cases of incontinence remained untreated. Jordan (2007) found that health professionals often trivialised the problem, seeing it as normal for older women to 'leak' or 'dribble'. Jordan also found that management of incontinence was usually 'conservative' consisting of behaviour training which emphasised that the woman was responsible for regaining control over her bladder; this could lead to women being denied access to potentially successful medical interventions. Her interviews with health professionals suggested that they could often make negative moral judgements about patients who found it difficult to exercise control over their bladder. Mitteness and Barker (1995) have also suggested that incontinence can profoundly damage an individual's identity. They found that incontinence could often lead health and social care professionals to judge an older person as no longer a 'proper adult'. Health and social care professionals frequently saw incontinence as indicative of a loss of 'self-control' rather than as a physical problem. These negative judgements could ultimately lead to institutionalisation. These judgemental attitudes among professionals make it unsurprising that people with incontinence are often reluctant to seek help and continue to hide it.

REFLECTION POINT

We have seen in this section that culturally ingrained rules governing conduct and manners place a particular value on the containment and concealment of bodily functions. As a result, people who experience a loss of control over bodily functions may experience a sense of shame and loss of dignity. They may also experience blame and social rejection.

As a health professional, reflect on your own experience of dealing with incontinent patients. Did you ever experience feelings of distaste or disgust? Did you ever feel that the patient should be able to exercise more control over their bladder or bowels? Did you ever assume that an elderly incontinent patient must also be mentally impaired?

Think about how you might challenge your own assumptions about the incontinent patient. How might you care for such patients with compassion while preserving their dignity and autonomy?

Disciplined Bodies

In this section we are going to consider the ways in which populations are disciplined and controlled through practices designed to control their bodies. We will be looking particularly at the work of a social historian called Michel Foucault. We can see Foucault's work as following a tradition in the social sciences which has been described as 'critical theory'.

The term **critical theory** is used to describe those approaches in the social sciences which are concerned with inequality and the ways in which those in power create structures, belief systems and practices which allow them to maintain dominance and control. An important founding group of critical theorists were the Frankfurt School, established in 1923, who wrote critically about the rise of Nazism. A key critical theorist and successor to the Frankfurt School was the German philosopher Jurgen Habermas. The term *critical theory* is used to apply to any approach which is focused on revealing and critically examining power structures. A particular focus in critical theory is the analysis of ideologies and discourses which support and justify domination and inequality in society. Examples of critical theory approaches include feminist theory, neo-Marxist theory, critical race theory, postcolonial theory and structuralism (Buchanan, 2018).

The work of Michel Foucault has been influential in critical theory because of his focus on the relationship between power and knowledge. However, he differs from many critical theorists in that he is regarded as a 'poststructuralist' who is concerned with the 'micro-politics' of power in everyday practices rather than with power structures. He was sceptical about the existence of social structures instead seeing power as a diffuse system of micro powers exercised in ordinary life. A key concept in his work is 'discourse' which describes ways of thinking underpinned by taken-for-granted assumptions (Ritzer, 2008). Critics of this poststructuralist approach have argued that it overplays the importance of discourse in the creation of conforming and compliant populations and downplays the continued use of force and coercion by institutions holding power. It also ignores the ways in which systems of social control function to perpetuate social inequalities (Garrett, 2020). We will look at Foucault's ideas about the exercise of power in relation to the body next.

Michel Foucault (1926–1984) was a French social theorist and historian of ideas. His studies focused particularly on the relationship between power and forms of knowledge. He was interested in the ways in which new forms of knowledge were deployed in institutions to discipline and control populations. One of his key concepts was 'governmentality' which described the ways in which institutions use 'techniques of the self' to induce people to internalise disciplinary controls and become 'self-governing subjects'. His historical studies of governmentality included histories of punishment, prisons, asylums and clinics. Of particular interest to health professionals are his history of madness (Madness and Civilisation, first published in 1960) and of medicine (The Birth of the Clinic, first published in 1963).

Foucault was particularly interested in discovering how modern forms of social control developed. Foucault says that pre-modern societies were governed by absolute rulers (kings, dictators) who ruled by force and disciplined the populace through torture and execution. Punishment of non-conformity or rebellion was often by execution designed as a public 'spectacle' in which the body of the offender was ritually desecrated by, for example hanging, drawing and quartering. This gruesome public spectacle was designed to intimidate the population (Foucault, 2019).

Foucault suggests that as the population grew and society became more complex the decline of these public spectacles (such as public hangings) occurred. Confinement in institutions was seen as a more humane and effective way to control and reform the abnormal, criminal and deviant. Thus, there was a rapid growth in institutions, such as prisons, orphanages and hospitals, throughout the nineteenth century (we examine these institutions further in Chapter 10). These institutions developed a range of techniques of control designed to discipline inmates and make lasting changes to their behaviour. These involved the close observation, measurement and direction of individual's bodies (Foucault, 2003, 2006). Foucault suggests that this system of discipline, which originally developed to control inmate populations, developed gradually into a system of control that spread across the whole of society (Foucault, 2019). Foucault was one of a number of authors preoccupied with the social control functions of medicine. He saw healthcare as one of a number of institutions which schooled the population to conform to the rules of a bureaucratically ordered society.

The first thing to say about the development of this system of discipline was that it focused on individuals and involved very detailed examination of their behaviour. Foucault described three key techniques which he saw as central to this new disciplinary regime which diffused through society.

- **Hierarchical observation:** Within institutions, such as prisons, inmates were subject to continuous surveillance so they would be aware at all times that they could be watched. For example, prisons had central watch towers to oversee inmates and spyholes in individual cells. Foucault called this all-seeing eye the 'panoptican'. This type of observation also involved keeping detailed records of the person being watched. An example today would be CCTV surveillance of workplaces or schools to regulate behaviours, such as frequency of toilet breaks. This constant inspecting gaze is designed to convince the individual that they need to start to regulate their own behaviour by instilling the constant fear of being watched, found out and punished. Foucault suggests that gradually these fears are internalised until individuals become self-policing (Foucault, 2019).
- Secondly, **normalising judgement** involves individuals' being repeatedly measured, assessed and compared to others. This system of measurement allows yardsticks (norms) for judging normality, such as the tests used on children to determine whether their physical and mental development is normal. A variety of professions may be charged with the task of judging normality, such as psychiatrists, teachers and social workers (Foucault, 2019). In the workplace, systems of audit, inspection and appraisal perform the same function and instil a fear of being judged as performing below the norm.
- The final instrument of discipline described by Foucault is the **examination.** This involves the individual being both assessed and corrected. This combines observation and normalising judgement into what Foucault calls the **'normalising gaze'**. The examination relies on **objectifying** the individual. It requires the professional to set aside any human sympathies and defer to an impersonal measurement system. This objectifying gaze in turn allows the individual to be disposed of into a particular category. It might, for example, allow them to qualify for a 'better' school or be selected for a 'special' school for the 'learning disabled'. It might also determine whether they are considered to have defects in need of correction; for example, a badly behaved school child might be declared to be acting 'abnormally' and thus a candidate for drug treatment for 'attention deficit hyperactivity disorder' (Foucault, 2019).

For Foucault, there were a number of key points to notice about disciplinary power. Firstly, it is impersonal. It is not imposed from the top by powerful individuals; it is instead diffused throughout society and wide networks of people are involved in its exercise; not only formal occupations, such as doctors and teachers who make judgements about others and enforce norms, but parents, neighbours etc. Secondly, its success depends on the creation of the 'self-disciplining' subject who internalises social norms and becomes self-policing. Thus, according to Foucault, disciplinary power has become less obvious and intrusive over time as it has become incorporated into everyday life, while self-control and self-management have become central values in society. There are new challenges in the 'information age' as the capacity for surveillance has dramatically increased and we will consider these later. Firstly, we will consider an example of disciplinary power in action by looking at attitudes towards those considered to deviate from a normal body weight.

OBESITY, WEIGHT STIGMA AND VICTIM BLAMING

The World Health Organization defines obesity as 'abnormal or excessive fat accumulation that may impair health' (WHO, 2020). It estimates that 39% of adults worldwide are overweight and 13% are obese (WHO, 2020). Obesity is defined by a measure called the body mass index (BMI). It took some time for the BMI to be widely accepted as the standard measure of what constituted 'normal' or 'abnormal' body weight (Fletcher, 2014). The WHO defines a BMI of over 30 as indicative of obesity while a BMI of 25+ indicates a person is overweight. These norms were debated over several decades before agreement was reached and thus a BMI between 25 and 30 that we define as 'overweight' today was often considered normal in the 1970s. We can see the development of this standard measure as the development and gradual hardening of what Foucault (2019) would call **'normalising judgement'**.

Running alongside the establishment of the BMI as a standard measure was the increasing involvement of psychiatry in redefining obesity as a failure of self-control rather than a problem of metabolism (Rasmussen, 2012). Rasmussen links this to tensions in post-war consumerist culture which both offered a consumerist paradise of unlimited consumption and yet, at the same time, wanted to restrain consumption and 'overindulgence' in order to reinforce social norms of hard work, self-discipline and conformity. As social perceptions of the causes of obesity hardened, this had implications for attitudes towards people considered overweight.

A study by the World Obesity Forum (2018) found that stigma and discrimination against people considered overweight was a global issue. They described weight stigma as negative behaviours and attitudes directed at people purely because of their weight. Their study focused on the media and identified a wealth of negative messages portraying the obese as lazy, greedy, lacking willpower and unattractive. Typically, in news items on obesity, the media shows us shots of headless obese people walking in the street. The camera focuses on their abdomen or buttocks and on areas of protruding flesh. We are not being shown a human being with whom we could sympathise but a faceless personification of fatness. We are invited to judge and to objectify (Puhl et al., 2013). Lupton (2015) suggests that these media images are designed to evoke negative moral and aesthetic judgements and, more particularly, to stimulate feelings of disgust towards the obese.

We introduced the concept of stigma in Chapter 2 and discuss it in depth in Chapter 7. Goffman (2009) said **stigma** described the situation of the person who was 'disqualified' from social acceptance. When we stigmatise people we no longer see them as individuals. Instead, we stereotype them as simply members of a category to which we have assigned negative characteristics. In the case of obesity, we stereotype obese people by inferring negative character traits, such as laziness, greed and lack of willpower. We considered poverty stigma in Chapter 2 and there is evidence suggesting that poverty and weight stigma frequently intersect. Stigma can result in discrimination and social rejection and can also be internalised leading to depression, loss of confidence and shame. It has thus been suggested that weight stigma is counterproductive, making it more difficult for individuals to lose weight (Jackson et al., 2014). Weight stigma can also intersect with other forms of prejudice and discrimination as we saw in the case of poverty. Thus, according to Ciciurkaite and Perry (2018), the wealthy are to some degree insulated from weight stigma whereas the less affluent and those from ethnic minorities experience greater stigma.

According to Saguy and Almeling (2008), public health professionals have encouraged public prejudice against the obese. Using Foucault's terminology we could say they have encouraged both **hierarchical observation** and **normalising judgement**. Couch et al., (2018) have noted how public health campaigns on obesity, such as the Australian 'LiveLighter' campaign, invoked fear and disgust by referring to body fat as 'toxic' and showing graphic images of surgically opened bodies with the visceral fat displayed. More importantly, public health campaigns have presented obesity as a 'preventable' illness and simplified the issue of obesity to a matter of individual willpower, ignoring the complex web of social factors that have led to a rise in obesity (Couch et al., 2018, Saguy & Almeling, 2008). These include the rise in sedentary occupations, long working hours, the aggressive marketing of ultra-processed, fast foods high in fat, salt and sugar, and the increase in food poverty. Lupton (2015) describes this approach to health promotion as the 'pedagogy of disgust' and says it is unethical and counterproductive.

In a classic paper, Crawford (1980) described the rise of what he called **'healthism'** in the post-war era. He said health had been elevated to a 'super value' in Western societies imposing a moral responsibility on individuals to be health conscious and to feel personally responsible for the health of their bodies. Health and ill health are no longer seen as states that we enjoy or suffer through no fault of our own. Health has become central to self-identity and something we are held personally responsible for achieving. People are morally judged by 'how well they succeed or fail in adopting healthy practices' (Crawford, 2006, p. 402). We are required to constantly police our own bodies and engage with projects for self-improvement, such as diets and online work-outs. As a result, ill health is judged as resulting from weakness of character as we have seen in the example of weight stigma above. Crawford said this deflected attention from the economic, political and social causes of ill health allowing people to **'blame the victim'** for their own health while promoting self-blame among the ill (see Chapter 1).

Healthism also commits the health-conscious to what Crawford calls a 'spiral of control and anxiety'. Being health conscious and engaging in healthy behaviour should make us feel more secure about our health, but the media continually brings new health threats to our attention thus creating new health anxieties. We can link both 'healthism', 'victim blaming' and 'weight stigma' back to Foucault's concept of disciplinary power. Both involve attempts to impose a **normalising gaze** in order to exercise control over individual behaviours. In particular, both reinforce the demand that individuals internalise normalising judgements (for example, by worrying about their weight) and exercise a high degree of control over their bodily functions.

REFLECTION POINT: WEIGHT STIGMA

Think about your own observations of positive and negative images of fat and thin individuals in the media. How have these images and the messages they convey made you feel about your own body size and shape?

Now think about your own attitudes to patients who are overweight or obese. What assumptions and judgements have you made about these people? How do you think these may have affected the patients you were caring for?

IDENTITY AND BODY PROJECTS

We have seen in the preceding sections that bodily self-control and self-improvement are central values in modern society. As a result, the image our body presents has become the primary way in which our identity is evaluated; a contemporary example of this is the ritualised presentation of the self to others through online posting of 'selfies'(Faimau, 2020). As we noted earlier, our body and its appearance is no longer seen as something we are born with and should accept. We are increasingly encouraged to work on and modify our bodies in order to project an image that matches the self-identity that we desire. Bodies may be modified for a variety of reasons; to signify membership of a particular social group; to signify a change in social status or to conform to prevailing aesthetic standards of physical attractiveness (Featherstone, 2000). A growing number of technologies to modify the body, such as implants and prosthetics, are commercially promoted.

One type of body modification which has been on the increase in recent decades is practices which permanently mark the body, such as tattooing and piercing. In traditional societies body markings signified membership of a group, a life cycle transition or a change in social status and were often obligatory. An example is traditional Maori tattoos. Turner (1999) suggests that tattoos are now more closely linked to 'the commercial exploitation of sexual themes in popular culture'. Today, Turner (1999) suggests, people obtain body marks to express their individuality. Tattoos can be highly personal but can just be designed to look fashionable and 'cool'. Turner sees them as a sign of the individualism of modern society. This contrasts with traditional societies where body marks signified a collective identity.

This raises the question as to why people in contemporary society are more disposed to mark or change their bodies permanently to express individual identity. Shilling (1993) has suggested that the body's appearance has become a much more significant marker of identity in contemporary culture. He draws on the work of Giddens (1991) who argued that life in fast-paced, modern societies is dominated by feelings of risk and insecurity. The body has become the one thing over which individuals feel they may be able to exercise some control to alleviate these feelings of insecurity. As a result, our bodies can often become the focus of **'body projects'**. These can involve attempts to maintain a slim, fit and healthy body or attempts to alter its size, shape or appearance. Shilling (1993) suggests that we may feel compelled to engage in these 'body projects' because the dominant culture places particular value on particular body forms (as we have seen in the case of weight stigma). Body projects can improve health and make people feel good about themselves. However, they can also make people feel even more insecure, unsuccessful or stigmatised. In addition, they can sometimes involve health-damaging modifications to the body, such as extreme dieting. Cultural values can change quite rapidly in modern consumer culture, leading people to feel continuing insecurities about their bodies (Featherstone, 2000). Note the similarities here to the 'spiral of control and anxiety' described by Crawford (2006).

Reischer and Koo (2004) suggest that the main reason that individuals modify their bodies is to try to live up to changing standards of beauty. They note, for example, that even Barbie had to go 'under the knife', being reshaped in 1997 to fit changing norms about female body shape. Whilst traditionally maintaining a 'beautiful' body, which is carefully controlled in size and appearance, was an expectation imposed mainly on women in contemporary society, men too have come under pressure, with an enormous increase in body maintenance products marketed to men.

We see the increase in attempts to modify the body to fit a cultural ideal most clearly in the rise in cosmetic surgery and other invasive procedures, such as liposuction, 'fillers' and Botox injections. Cosmetic surgery has become a multi-billion pound industry. Elliott (2011) suggests that it has been promoted in popular culture through phenomena, such as TV makeover shows, glossy magazines and celebrity culture. In particular, these media have sold the message that body modification is the route to happiness and life satisfaction. Elliott argues that celebrity culture has moved away from a focus on celebrity personalities and talents towards a focus on celebrities' bodies and specifically on their body parts. He suggests that the media often encourages us to deconstruct and objectify celebrity bodies by, for example, admiring (or criticising) Kim Kardashian's buttocks, Angelie Jolie's lips or Liz Hurley's bust. He notes that requests for cosmetic surgery are now often framed in terms of requests to copy the body parts of individual celebrities. It is hard to avoid the conclusion that celebrity culture has played a significant role in increasing people's insecurities about their bodies. As a result there has been considerable criticism of the impact of celebrity culture on people's psychological well-being and its role in promoting 'body dissatisfaction' (Grogan, 2021).

DIGITAL TECHNOLOGIES AND THE SURVEILLANCE OF BODIES

We will now briefly consider the impact of digital technologies on individuals' relationships with their bodies. The smartphone is now carried in the pockets of around 80% of the UK population who spend on average between two and three hours per day using their phones. Almost half of these smartphone users regularly post 'selfies' on social media. In addition, it has been estimated that at least one-quarter of the population own some type of wearable fitness tracker (Ofcom, 2018). Fitness apps allow the continuous quantification of various features of bodily health, such as vital signs, as well as monitoring and quantifying daily activities, such as number of steps walked, hours slept and calories ingested. These various devices enroll individual users into a continuous self-improvement project in which they learn to engage with constant self-surveillance over their bodily appearance, health and health behaviours (Ajana, 2017). These self-tracking behaviours have been described as the quantification of the self (Lupton, 2013). Through self-tracking we learn to think about our bodies in terms of numbers and metrics which measure our performance against set standards. Some authors have seen these monitoring techniques as clear proof that we have internalised the **'normalising gaze'** described by Foucault (Simon, 2005).

Others have noted the dark side to these technologies as they intensify control by the state and corporations just as much as they facilitate self-control. For example, wearable trackers are increasingly used by employers, such as Amazon, to microscopically control their workers actions thus raising ethical and privacy issues (Ajana, 2017). In an extreme form of this type of surveillance some firms in Sweden and the United States have begun to microchip employees with tracking technologies than can be neither removed nor turned off (Kollewe, 2018). The use of fitness tracking technologies by employers allows them to monitor employees' health in ways that invade their right to privacy and can be discriminatory (Brassart Olsen, 2020). These trends have been seen by some as indicative of the rise of a surveillance society, which has frightening implications for human freedoms, potentially allowing whole populations to be subject to minute-to-minute state or corporate surveillance (Zuboff, 2019).

Like the other body projects we have discussed, self-tracking has the potential to give people a sense of control over their health; for example, it is widely used by athletes to improve their performance. However, it also has the potential to increase anxiety and body dissatisfaction and to subject the individual to intensified control by commercial and state institutions. Thus, its wider ethical and political implications have yet to be fully realised.

REFLECTION POINT: SELF-TRACKING

Have you used a fitness tracker or smart watch to monitor your own health and health behaviours? What do you think are the positive and negative effects of these technologies?

New developments in healthcare, such as the 'virtual ward', require patients to use digital tracking technologies to monitor their health at home. What do you think the positive and negative implications of these developments are for patients' privacy, autonomy, wellbeing and safety?

Summary of Key Points

- Our understanding of our body is influenced by culture, subjective experience and our interactions with others.
- Contemporary society places a high cultural value on the control of bodily functions as a result of what Elias called the 'civilising process'. This can have negative social consequences for people suffering from conditions that impair their control of bodily functions, such as leaking wounds and incontinence.
- Michel Foucault suggested that contemporary society strictly controls and regulates bodies as part of a system of institutional knowledge which is used to control populations. He saw this as the principle way in which power is exercised in contemporary society. An example of this regulation of bodies is the promotion of weight stigma.
- In contemporary society, people are frequently encouraged to be dissatisfied with their bodies and to modify them by 'body projects', such as slimming and cosmetic surgery. This can have negative implications for people's wellbeing.

Further Reading

Elliott, A. (2011). 'I want to look like that!' Cosmetic surgery and celebrity culture. *Cultural Sociology, 5*(4), 463–477.
Helman, C. (2007). *Culture, health and illness.* CRC press.
Lawton, J. (1998). Contemporary hospice care: The sequestration of the unbounded body and 'dirty dying'. *Sociology of Health & Illness, 20*(2), 121–143.

Lupton, D. (2015). The pedagogy of disgust: The ethical, moral and political implications of using disgust in public health campaigns. *Critical Public Health, 25*(1), 4–14.

Twigg, J. (2011). *The body in health and social care*. Macmillan International.

References

Ajana, B. (2017). Digital health and the biopolitics of the Quantified Self. *Digital Health, 3*, 1–18.

Baer, R. D., Weller, S. C., de Alba García J. G., & Salcedo Rocha, A. L. (2008). Cross-cultural perspectives on physician and lay models of the common cold. *Medical Anthropology Quarterly, 22*(2), 148–166.

Bourdieu, P. (2013). *Outline of a theory of practice*. Cambridge University Press.

Bourdieu, P., Accardo, A., & Emanuel, S. (1999). *The weight of the world: Social suffering in contemporary society*. John Wiley and Sons Ltd.

Boyle, C. M., (1970). Difference between patients' and doctors' interpretation of some common medical terms. *BMJ, 2*(5704), 286–289.

Brassart Olsen C. (2020). To track or not to track? Employees' data privacy in the age of corporate wellness, mobile health, and GDPR. *International Data Privacy Law, 10*(3), 236–252.

Buchanan, I. (2018). *A dictionary of critical theory*. Oxford University Press.

Carter, S.K., (2010). Beyond control: Body and self in women's childbearing narratives. *Sociology of Health & Illness, 32*(7), 993–1009.

Ciciurkaite, G, & Perry, B. L. (2018). Body weight, perceived weight stigma and mental health among women at the intersection of race/ethnicity and socioeconomic status: Insights from the modified labelling approach. *Sociology of Health & Illness, 40*(1), 18–37.

Couch, D., Fried, A., & Komesaroff, P. (2018). Public health and obesity prevention campaigns—A case study and critical discussion. *Communication Research and Practice, 4*(2), 149–166.

Crawford, R. (1980). Healthism and the medicalization of everyday life. *International Journal of Health Services, 10*(3), 365–388.

Crawford, R. (2006). Health as a meaningful social practice. *Health, 10*(4), 401–420.

Douglas, M. (2003). *Purity and danger: An analysis of concepts of pollution and taboo*. Routledge.

Elias, N. (2012). *The civilizing process*. Blackwell.

Elliott, A. (2011). 'I want to look like that!' Cosmetic surgery and celebrity culture. *Cultural Sociology, 5*(4), 463–477.

Faimau, G. (2020). Towards a theoretical understanding of the selfie: A descriptive review. *Sociology Compass, 14*(12), 1–12.

Featherstone, M. (2000). *Body modification: An introduction*. Sage Publications.

Fletcher, I. (2014). Defining an epidemic: The body mass index in British and US obesity research 1960–2000. *Sociology of Health & Illness, 36*(3), 338–353.

Foucault, M. (2003). *The birth of the clinic* (3rd ed.). Routledge.

Foucault, M. (2019). *Discipline & punish: The birth of the prison*. Penguin Books.

Foucault, M. (2006). *Madness and civilization*. Vintage Books.

Garrett, P. M., (2020). Faulty 'tools'? Why social work scholarship needs to take a more critical approach to Michel Foucault. *Journal of Social Work, 20*(4), 483–500.

Giddens, A. (1991). *Modernity and self-identity: Self and society in the late modern age*. Stanford University Press.

Goffman, E. (2009). *Stigma: Notes on the management of spoiled identity*. Penguin Books.

Gottlieb, A. (2020). Menstrual taboos: Moving beyond the curse. In C. Bobel, I. T. Winkler, B. Fahs, K. A. Hasson, E. A. Kissling & T. A. Roberts (Eds.), *The palgrave handbook of critical menstruation studies* (pp. 143–162). Palgrave Macmillan.

Greenhalgh, T., Helman, C., & Chowdhury, A. (1998). Health beliefs and folk models of diabetes in British Bangladeshis: A qualitative study (long version). *British Medical Journal, 316*, 978–983.

Grogan, S. (2021). *Body image: Understanding body dissatisfaction in men, women and children*. Taylor & Francis.

Helman, C. (2007). *Culture, health and illness*. CRC Press.

Helman, C. G., (1978). Feed a cold, starve a fever"—Folk models of infection in an English suburban community, and their relation to medical treatment. *Culture, Medicine and Psychiatry, 2*(2), 107–137.

Jackson, S. E., Beeken, R. J., & Wardle, J. (2014). Perceived weight discrimination and changes in weight, waist circumference, and weight status. *Obesity, 22*(12), 2485–2488.

Jordan, J. (2007). Containing the 'leaky' body: Female urinary incontinence and formal health care. In M. Kirkham (Ed.), *Exploring the dirty side of women's health* (pp. 206–218). Routledge.

Kollewe J. (2018). Alarm over talks to implant UK employees with microchips. *The Guardian*. Retrieved November 11, 2018, from https://www.theguardian.com/technology/2018/nov/11/alarm-over-talks-to-implant-uk-employees-with-microchips.

Lawler, J. (2006). *Behind the Screens: Nursing, somology, and the problem of the body*. Sydney University Press.

Lawton, J. (1998). Contemporary hospice care: The sequestration of the unbounded body and 'dirty dying. *Sociology of Health & Illness, 20*(2), 121–143.

Linklater, A., & Mennell, S. (2010). Norbert Elias, the civilizing process: Sociogenetic and psychogenetic investigations—An overview and assessment. *History and Theory, 49*(3), 384–411.

Lupton, D. (2013). Quantifying the body: Monitoring and measuring health in the age of mHealth technologies. *Critical Public Health, 23*(4), 393–403.

Lupton, D. (2015). The pedagogy of disgust: The ethical, moral and political implications of using disgust in public health campaigns. *Critical Public Health, 25*(1), 4–14.

Mittenese, L. S., & Barker, J. C. (1995). Stigmatizing a "normal" condition: Urinary incontinence in late life. *Medical Anthropology Quarterly, 9*(2), 188–210.

Nettleton, S. (2006). *The sociology of health and illness*. Polity Press.

Ofcom. (2018). *The communications market report*. https://www.ofcom.org.uk/research-and-data/multi-sector-research/cmr/cmr-2018/interactive.

Peake, S, & Manderson, L. (2003). The constraints of a normal life: The management of urinary incontinence by middle aged women. *Women & Health, 37*(3), 37–51.

Poku, B. A., Caress, A. L., & Kirk, S. (2020). Body as a machine": How Adolescents with sickle cell disease construct their fatigue experiences. *Qualitative Health Research, 30*(9), 1431–1444.

Porter, R. (2003). *Blood and guts: A short history of medicine*. Penguin Books.

Prior, L, Evans, M. R., & Prout, H. (2011). Talking about colds and flu: The lay diagnosis of two common illnesses among older British people. *Social Science & Medicine, 73*(6), 922–928.

Puhl, R. M., Peterson, J. L., DePierre, J. A., & Luedicke, J. (2013). Headless, hungry, and unhealthy: A video content analysis of obese persons portrayed in online news. *Journal of Health Communication, 18*(6), 686–702.

Rasmussen, N. (2012). Weight stigma, addiction, science, and the medication of fatness in mid-twentieth century America. *Sociology of Health & Illness, 34*(6), 880–895.

Reischer, E., & Koo., K. S. (2004). The body beautiful: Symbolism and agency in the social world. *Annual Review of Anthropology, 33*, 297–317.

Ritzer, G. (2008). *Sociological theory*. McGraw Hill.

Saguy, A. C., & Almeling, R. (2008). Fat in the fire? Science, the news media, and the "obesity epidemic". *Sociological Forum, 23*(1), 53–83.

Shilling, C. (1993). *The body and social theory*. Sage Publications.

Simon, B. (2005). The return of panopticism: Supervision, subjection and the new surveillance. *Surveillance & Society, 3*(1), 1–20.

Turner, B. S. (1999). The possibility of primitiveness: Towards a sociology of body marks in cool societies. *Body & Society, 5*(2–3), 39–50.

Twigg, J. (2011). *The body in health and social care*. Macmillan International.

Weinman, J, Yusuf, G., Berks, R., Rayner, S., & Petrie, K. J. (2009). How accurate is patients' anatomical knowledge: A cross-sectional, questionnaire study of six patient groups and a general public sample. *BMC Family Practice, 10*(1), 1–6.

World Health Organisation. (2020). *Obesity and overweight factsheet*. Retrieved January 08, 2024, from. https://www.who.int/en/news-room/fact-sheets/detail/obesity-and-overweight.

World Obesity Forum. (2018). *Weight stigma in the media*. https://www.worldobesity.org/resources/resource-library/world-obesity-day-2018-media-report.

Zuboff, S. (2019). *The age of surveillance capitalism: The fight for a human future at the new frontier of power*. Profile Books.

CHAPTER 6

Concepts of Health and Illness and the Illness Experience

The introduction to this book discussed the differences between social and biomedical models of health and illness. This chapter picks up these arguments again and looks in more detail at how medical and 'lay' conceptions of illness differ. The chapter will look at how social institutions and culture influence both medical and 'lay' conceptions of health and illness, causing both to change over time and to vary between different cultures. It will also look at the ways in which definitions of ill health have changed over time through processes that have been described as 'medicalisation' and 'demedicalisation'.

The chapter will then explore how people seek help with periods of illness and how they subjectively experience illness and its meaning. It will explore the difficulties that arise from the mismatch in understandings of health and illness between the public and health professionals. It will also examine what happens when people seek help; here it will consider diagnosis as a social process occurring within an institutional context. It will also look at communication problems in the diagnostic process and consider why certain groups of people find it very difficult to get a diagnosis despite having the signs and symptoms of a medically recognised condition. This will lead to a discussion about how consultations between patients and health professionals are influenced by social and cultural factors. Finally, the chapter will consider how the experience of being ill can be affected by negative moral judgements about people who are sick. This issue will be discussed further in the chapter on long-term illness and disability.

Concepts of Health and Illness

WHAT IS HEALTH?

Sociologists have been interested for many years in how different groups define health. What do we mean when we say we are healthy and how do we decide that we are no longer healthy but are ill? Definitions of health have also had political significance, since governments are frequently judged on the impact of their actions on the health of their population. Thus, in an ambitious political statement the constitution of the World Health Organization stated that:

> *'Health is a state of complete physical, mental and social well-being and not merely the absence of disease or infirmity. The enjoyment of the highest attainable standard of health is one of the fundamental rights of every human being without distinction of race, religion, political belief, economic or social condition.'*

(WHO, 1946)

This definition of health is a product of the discipline of public health (see Chapter 1). It is an aspirational definition which could leave many of us defined as ill for much of the time. Although there are benefits to aspiring to achieve positive health for populations, the definition has been criticised and described as an invitation to the overmedicalisation of populations (Crawford, 1980). How we define health is of interest both to sociologists and clinicians. This is because how we define health influences our expectations of our health and, consequently, our decisions about when to seek help. Do you accept tiredness, aches and pains or feelings of sadness as normal for someone of your age and situation, or do you expect a higher level of well-being and seek medical help? We will look at how people make these decisions later.

Sociologists have been interested to find out what ideas and expectations of health are shared by the general population and to what extent differences in culture and social conditions impact how people define health. Sociologists have distinguished a number of key ideas about health which have to some extent crossed cultures and social groups. People's ideas about health are complex and may change over time. Most people will hold a mixture of different ideas about what constitutes good health. Blaxter (2003) carried out a study in Scotland to investigate people's conceptions of health. She identified a number of key ideas which were expressed by participants.

Examples: 'Lay' Concepts of Health

- Health is not being ill: *'He's never seen a doctor in 50 years'* (p. 20)
- Health is being able to function: *'She's 81 … and she does the garden'* (p. 28)
- Health is a reserve capacity: *'He belongs to healthy stock'* (p. 23)
- Health is fitness and vitality: *'I can do something strenuous and don't feel tired'* (p. 24)
- Health is psychosocial well-being: *'Emotionally you are stable energetic happier and things don't bother you'* (p. 29)
- Health is good social relationships: *'I enjoy life more and can work and help other people'* (p. 27)
- Health is leading a 'healthy life': *'I call her healthy because she goes jogging and doesn't eat fried food'* (p. 23) Blaxter (2003).

We can see that there are a range of ideas about what it means to be healthy. Blaxter found that people's conceptions of what it means to be healthy change across the life course with older people placing less stress on physical fitness. She also found some differences in men and women's ideas about health, with women placing more emphasis on social relationships. She found only minor differences related to social class (Blaxter, 2003). Macintyre et al. (2006) made similar findings. Both studies were conducted in the West of Scotland, so the ethnic diversity of their study population was limited. Some studies have shown some limited ethnic variations in concepts of health, although in the past these have been overstated (Ahmad & Bradby, 2007). Thus, despite some differences, there are many similarities in the concepts of health held by different demographic groups.

As we saw in the previous chapter, people's ideas about their bodies and bodily health are affected by their lifeworld as well as by the wider culture around them, including the culture of biomedicine. Before we consider people's experience of illness, we will look again at the biomedical model of illness which is central to the diagnosis and treatment of individual patients.

THE BIOMEDICAL MODEL

As we noted in the introduction, the biomedical model has been described as a reductionist model which focuses on the biological basis of illness. It conceives of health narrowly as an absence of disease. Disease itself is normally determined by the identification of specific biological changes. Thus, medicine distinguishes **'symptoms'** (indications of an illness as experienced by the patient, such as pain, fatigue or nausea) from clinical **'signs'** of illness (indications of illness as observed by a clinician through examination or tests). Signs are often presumed by health professionals to be 'objective' evidence of disease while 'symptoms' are often regarded as subjective and thus unreliable indicators of illness by clinicians. In the case of psychiatric diagnosis, biological markers of illness rarely exist, so psychiatric diagnosis still depends on an analysis of symptoms and behaviours. However, the biological basis of symptoms is still assumed, and the psychiatrist's observations are often privileged over patients' reports of symptoms (Brown, 1990).

The biomedical model also employs a mechanistic model of health, often treating the body like a machine that can be repaired. Thus, going to the doctor can be compared to taking the car into the garage to be fixed (see Chapter 10). The medical 'garage' then offers a narrow menu of technical solutions mainly involving drugs or surgery. Nettleton (2021), however, suggests that technological solutions to illness may be overplayed, since this model of illness separates the person from their body. This means it ignores the social factors in a person's life which have contributed to illness. At the same time, it disregards the subjective meanings of illness as experienced by the patient.

Freund et al., (2003) suggest that the biomedical model gives priority to precisely classifying diseases. The medical model incorporates the idea of **'disease specificity'**, that is, the belief that every disease or syndrome can and should be tightly defined by a specific list of signs and symptoms. This belief in 'disease specificity' can lead to academic argument and debate over disease classifications which may be frequently revised. For example, the autoimmune disease, systemic lupus erythematosus (or lupus), which mainly affects women, has several rival classification systems all of which have been subject to revisions. This may have real consequences for patients. As we saw in Chapter 3, in the case of lupus, diagnosis takes on average almost 7 years from first presentation of symptoms (Sloan et al., 2020). We will return to the process of diagnosis and the factors affecting it later in the chapter. Firstly, we will look at how categories of medical 'disorders' have been expanding since the mid-twentieth century in a process that has been described as 'medicalisation'.

Changing Definitions of Illness: Medicalisation

Sociologists and political theorists have taken a particular interest in the expansion of medical diagnoses and this process of expansion has been called 'medicalisation'. Medicalisation refers, firstly, to the process through which a variety of life's problems and discomforts get newly defined as medical disorders and, secondly, it refers to the growing influence of different types of medical authority on our lives. The expansion of medical disorders has taken a number of forms. This has included:

- Redefining ordinary biological processes, such as puberty or the menopause, as medical problems
- Redefining unhappy experiences, such as grief, as medical disorders
- Redefining 'problem' behaviours, such as 'hyperactivity' in children as medical disorders.

There has been rapid growth in diagnostic categories since the mid-twentieth century. Sociologists have seen this as indicating the growing medicalisation of human problems and differences (Conrad & Barker, 2010). In particular, medicine has significantly expanded into the management of behavioural, psychological and social problems. For example, the Diagnostic and Statistical Manual of Mental Disorders (DSM) produced by the American Psychiatric Association is widely used to diagnose mental illness. Since the first version of DSM was published in 1952, there have been five editions, and the number of mental disorders defined by DSM has increased from 106 in the first edition to approximately 541 in DSM-5 published in 2013 (Blashfield et al., 2014). As the DSM has developed, there have been some controversial additions to its classification system. For example, shyness used to be seen as part of the normal range of human behaviours but, as a result of medicalisation, shyness can be labelled as 'social anxiety disorder'. According to Scott, this changes what was once a normal human experience into something pathological (Scott, 2006). Similarly, grief used to be seen as a normal reaction to loss, but has been redefined as a 'disorder' by DSM-5 if it lasts longer than 12 months.

Sociologists have suggested a variety of explanations for medicalisation and have drawn on different theoretical perspectives, such as social constructionism and critical theory, to inform their explanations. One of the earliest and simplest explanations of medicalisation was that it was due to increased professional dominance (see also Chapter 9). Friedson described this as **'medical imperialism'** (Freidson, 1970). He suggested that, like an imperial country, the medical profession was colonising territory formerly occupied by other professions, such as the police, the judiciary and the clergy. Behaviours once described as criminal or sinful now came under the jurisdiction of medicine, to be treated rather than punished. The rationale for this change was often that it resulted in a kinder and less judgemental approach to problems such as drug addiction and alcoholism. However, some of the early examples of medicalisation, such as medical treatment of homosexuality between the 1930s and 1970s, using techniques such as electric shock treatment and chemical castration, could scarcely have been described as more humane for patients (Dickinson et al., 2012). In the case of homosexuality, a process of demedicalisation took place as a result of sustained political campaigning. Homosexuality was originally listed as a 'sociopathic personality disorder' in the 1952 version of DSM. This label was removed from DSM-II in 1973, although it was replaced with the vaguer 'sexual orientation disorder' so, arguably, there has been some continued resistance to fully demedicalising homosexuality.

Another early writer on medicalisation was the Catholic theologian and philosopher Ivan Illich. In his book 'Medical Nemesis' (1975) he attacked modern medicine for causing harm to patients. He suggested that society was experiencing an epidemic of **'iatrogenesis'**; a word that means 'doctor caused sickness'. Illich suggested that there were three types of iatrogenesis. The first of these was **'clinical iatrogenesis'** which referred to the clinical damage that medicine could cause through medical errors, etc. The second was **'social iatrogenesis'**. Illich believed medicalisation was undermining individual autonomy by creating dependence on doctors and on drug treatments. Finally, Illich described **'cultural iatrogenesis'** as the loss of traditional ways of dealing with (and finding meaning in) pain, suffering and death. Illich was opposed to industrialisation and to modern institutions generally. He believed they undermined individual liberty. His critique of medicine reflected his libertarian conservatism which was often backward looking. Critics of Illich have suggested that he was nostalgic for a pre-industrial past that few of us would want to return to (Navarro, 1975). For example, he believed women's lives were better in the pre-industrial era, but few women would wish to go back to the levels of maternal and infant mortality which characterised this period. Nevertheless, his ideas have been very influential.

Zola (1972) suggested a number of social reasons for medicalisation and the increased influence of the medical profession. We can see his approach as broadly fitting within the tradition of critical theory. He believed that the medical profession was increasingly being called upon to exercise social control functions in contemporary societies. As a result, medicine was not only expanding categories of 'illness' but also pronouncing on a whole new range of human habits and behaviours. Everything from our sex lives to our hobbies could now be judged to be healthy or unhealthy. Medical prescriptions for how to live started to invade all areas of people's lives, telling people what to eat, how much to sleep, how much to exercise, etc. Crawford described this as 'the medicalisation of everyday life' (Crawford, 1980). Zola rejected the notion that this change was predominantly being driven by the medical profession. Instead, Zola believed that medicalisation resulted from the development of increasingly technocratic and bureaucratic societies which were expanding the social control of populations. He thought contemporary societies made growing demands on their populations to conform to bureaucratic standards of behaviour and performance in workplaces, schools, public places and in their private lives too. State institutions and corporations had increasingly turned to medicine to manage those whose performance and behaviours fell short. These people could then be medically 'helped' to fit in. We can see some similarities here to the concerns expressed in Foucault's work (see Chapter 5).

Conrad and Leiter (2004) agreed with Zola that medicalisation was not primarily due to the 'imperialism' of the medical profession. They cited the large commercial enterprises which had invested in promoting new and expanded medical labels, such as pharmaceutical and biotechnology firms. It has become increasingly common for these industries to market directly to the public using the media (and progressively, social media) to promote new medical labels for problems. This allows them to promote their products as cures for these 'new' illnesses. We saw this in the last chapter when we looked at the ways in which various industries have promoted body dissatisfaction.

This 'marketisation' of new illness labels is designed to promote consumer demand. Moynihan et al., (2002) have called this marketing of new medical conditions **'disease-mongering'** and note that 'there's a lot of money to be made from telling healthy people they are sick' (p. 886).

Example: 'Disease Mongering'

Drug companies in the US have committed enormous marketing resources to selling new disease labels both to health professionals and the public, allowing them to both brand and 'own' new diseases. The lack of regulation of 'direct to consumer' drug marketing in the US may be responsible for very high use of prescription drugs in the US. Ebeling describes how the drug company, Eli Lilly, campaigned to expand the sales of their anti-depressant drug Prozac by marketing it to premenstrual women. They began this campaign when their licence to market Prozac for depression was running out. The loss of this licence would allow doctors treating depression to substitute Prozac for a generic alternative. Thus, the company needed to look for a new market for Prozac. The company began a media campaign to market the new diagnostic label of Premenstrual Dysphoric Disorder (PMDD) direct to the public. This was described as a 'behavioural' disorder with emotional 'symptoms' which the campaign attributed to the premenstrual period. The campaign encouraged women to self-diagnose this 'new' condition, providing women with symptom checklists to promote self-diagnosis. At the same time, the company was working behind the scenes to promote official recognition of the condition and influence its official definition. The marketing of this diagnostic label then allowed Eli Lilly to apply for a licence to promote and sell Prozac for PMDD.

(EBELING, 2011)

There are some negative social consequences of medicalisation. These can include individuals being given unwanted medical labels (particularly in the mental health field); the unnecessary use of medication; the diversion of resources away from more serious illnesses; a waste of healthcare resources; encouraging health anxieties in the general public and putting too much emphasis on individual, drug-based solutions to personal and social problems (Moynihan et al., 2012).

Medicalisation has encouraged an expansion of medical categories, yet despite this, we know that most symptoms are not reported to a doctor but are self-managed at home (Calnan, 1987). We also know that some people have considerable difficulty getting a diagnosis (or a diagnosis is delayed) even though they are suffering from the signs and symptoms of a medically recognised condition (Sloan et al., 2020). In the next section, we will look at how potential patients make the decision to seek medical help and what difficulties they encounter when they do.

REFLECTION POINT: MEDICALISATION

Can you think of examples of 'new' medical conditions that you have come across in the media? What do you think the helpful and harmful effects of medicalisation might be?

The Experience of Illness

HELP-SEEKING AND THE JOURNEY TO DIAGNOSIS

We have already introduced the idea that people's cultural beliefs and what is happening in their lives influence how they perceive their bodies, as well as their ideas and expectations about their health. It should, therefore, come as no surprise to learn that people make decisions about when and where to seek medical help for symptoms with reference to what else is happening in their lives at the time.

In an early study, Zola (1973) suggested that symptoms, on their own, were often not enough to make people seek medical help. He described a number of '**triggers**' which led people to finally decide that it was now time to see a doctor. Triggers included:

- Symptoms interfering with physical or social activities, such as work or leisure
- Personal crises going on at the same time, such as a relationship breakdown
- Pressure from other people, such as family or employers, to seek help.

Zola also suggested that people 'temporalized' their symptoms. By this he meant that people set deadlines by deciding to wait until a certain time in the future in the hope that the illness would go away by itself. Other authors have noted that people tend to seek advice from a variety of other sources before seeking medical help. A study of a GP practice in Middlesbrough found that discussions with others were important to the decision to seek help for 70% of patients (Cornford & Cornford, 1999). Increasingly, people will also look to the internet as a source of information and advice (Nettleton et al., 2005). Informal advice may encourage or discourage people from seeking medical help. People may also try other remedies first, such as rest, home remedies and over-the-counter medicines, before seeking a medical consultation (Calnan, 1987).

Other factors that can affect help-seeking include the problem of fitting in a consultation around other life demands, for example work and family responsibilities. This can be particularly problematic for people in insecure, low-paid work, those with heavy caring responsibilities and others who lack sufficient time. The accessibility of services will also affect people's decisions. Unsurprisingly, long delays before receiving an appointment, long waits and difficult journeys to the nearest services can cause people to delay help-seeking, and these problems of access can disproportionately affect people from poorer backgrounds (Morgan & Thomas, 2009).

Freund et al., (2003) suggest that doctors and health systems make ambiguous and contradictory demands on patients. Patients are expected to get help for all 'genuine' medical conditions, particularly if they are 'serious'. They are also expected to know the 'right' place to present their problem. At the same time, patients must avoid 'bothering' the doctor with problems that are defined by doctors as 'trivial' or non-medical. Thus, on the one hand, patients are expected to have enough medical knowledge to know the difference between these two categories, yet at the same time within the consultation they are expected to defer to the doctor's 'expert' judgement. They are thus expected, on the one hand, to be an 'active expert' when making decisions about help-seeking while, on the other hand, to be 'humbly passive' once in the consultation room. This is something of a double-bind for patients and can lead to situations in which patients feel negatively judged by doctors.

There is evidence that past experiences with health services have an influence on delayed help-seeking. This is of particular concern when a person's fear of 'bothering' health professionals delays help-seeking for a serious illness such as cancer or heart disease. A review by Smith et al., (2005) of qualitative studies of diagnostic delay in cancer patients found that fear of being seen as a 'time-waster' or 'neurotic' was a significant deterrent to help-seeking for many patients, particularly when reinforced by family and friends. Coyle (1999) has suggested that **'personal identity threat'** is an important reason for dissatisfaction with healthcare and reluctance to engage with services. This included patients' feeling that they were not being treated as human beings. For patients, feeling dehumanised included the belief that their individual feelings, knowledge and experience had been devalued.

Coyle also suggests that the 'perspective difference' between patients and health professionals caused feelings of identity threat. Patients wanted their subjective feelings of pain and suffering to be recognised and acknowledged, whereas health professionals were interested in fitting their symptoms to a 'typical' case. Stereotyping of patients from different backgrounds, such as making ageist assumptions about older patients, was also a source of dissatisfaction (Coyle, 1999). Similarly, Malterud (2005) suggests that patients can suffer 'disempowering experiences of shame and humiliation' at the hands of health professionals. Malterud and Thesen (2008) suggest these are not deliberately inflicted but are unintended consequences. This often arises from the value placed on objectivity in medicine and the ways this can lead to an apparent dismissal of patients' concerns (Malterud, 2005). We will explore this issue more in the next section when we look at the process of diagnosis.

REFLECTION POINT

What should concern us most as healthcare practitioners are the impact of previous experiences of healthcare on people's subsequent decisions about help-seeking. What types of behaviour by health professionals might encourage or deter people from seeking help from healthcare services? What characteristics of healthcare institutions may create barriers to people seeking help?

THE EXPERIENCE OF DIAGNOSIS

In this section, we are going to look in a bit more detail at patients' experience of diagnosis. In order to understand how patients experience diagnosis we need first to consider how diagnosis has developed and changed as a social practice. According to one social historian (Jewson, 1976), there have been **three phases of medical knowledge**. The first phase was **'bedside medicine'**. This phase was linked to humoral medicine which we discussed in the previous chapter. Illness was diagnosed at the bedside and understood as both a physical and psychological disturbance of the whole person. Diagnosis was made largely by listening to the patient's narrative of their symptoms. In the second phase, which Jewson describes as **'hospital medicine'**, doctors came to rely more on physical examination of patients to detect signs of abnormality which they could correlate with specific diseases. The idea of disease specificity, which we mentioned earlier, developed, as did a clearer distinction between the patient's symptoms and clinical signs identified by the doctor. As a result, the patient's narrative of their symptoms became of diminishing importance to doctors who relied more on clinical examination. Finally, according to Jewson, **'laboratory medicine'** developed throughout the twentieth century. Doctors came to rely on laboratory tests more than physical examination. Increasingly, doctors felt there was no need to see or examine patients, and remote consultations became more common. Thus, diagnosis was increasingly determined by the results of tests conducted by laboratory workers at a distance from the patient.

If hospital medicine allowed doctors to stop listening to the patient's narrative, then laboratory medicine allowed them to stop looking at the patient, and instead to make their diagnosis whilst peering at a set of results in the patient's notes or on a computer screen. Laboratory medicine also moved power away from the bedside clinician and left less room for clinical judgement (see Chapter 9). Thresholds for diagnostic tests came to be decided by research and laboratory staff. Increasingly, diagnosis came to be governed by protocols laid down by remote bodies such as the National Institute for Care Excellence. Psychiatry has not been able to follow physical medicine into the laboratory but has established diagnostic criteria based on the observation of behaviours and symptoms. These have also been determined away from the bedside by guidelines and protocols created by expert panels of researchers and clinicians.

We will now think about the effects of these changes on the patient experience. Diagnosis 'legitimates' an illness, by which we mean that it gives it the status of something 'real' and gives the patient permission to be ill. This can have implications for patients on many levels. In particular, diagnosis is the gateway to treatment and care (Jutel, 2009). Recognition that a person is 'genuinely' ill is also important in relationships with family and friends as well as in more formal settings such as work, school, university and the benefits system. A diagnosis also reduces uncertainty, giving access to a treatment plan and some idea of the likely course of the illness. For the doctor, the diagnosis translates the illness as experienced by the patient into a 'disease' with a presumed biological basis, whilst also translating the patient from a person to a 'case' whose treatment will follow a specific treatment pathway. In contemporary healthcare, this pathway is often bureaucratically prescribed (Kleinman, 1988).

To achieve a diagnosis, doctors (and other health professionals, such as advanced practitioners) typically follow a decision tree which picks out what they determine as 'medically relevant' information from the patient's narrative in order to establish a pattern which fits a typical diagnostic category. The patient's narrative, however, is told in what the sociologist, Mishler (1984) describes as the **'voice of the lifeworld'** (see Chapter 5). This account typically includes an account of the circumstances in which the symptoms arose and then recounts the reasons for consultation; for example, that symptoms, such as pain and disability, are no longer manageable. Mishler describes the medical consultation as a process in which the **'voice of medicine'** continually interrupts the **'voice of the lifeworld'**, ignoring much of the patient's account and treating it as irrelevant 'noise', in order to impose a narrower, biomedical understanding of the patient's problem. This is done in order either to fit the patient into a known diagnostic category or to make a finding that evidence of disease is absent. This frequently has the effect of, firstly, ignoring the patient's concerns and, secondly, omitting from the medical account any contextual factors in the patient's life that have contributed to their ill health, such as domestic violence, poverty or a damaging working environment.

In addition, Freund et al., (2003) suggest that, despite its limitations, doctors do not simply impartially follow the biomedical model. Social influences can have a marked effect on medical decision-making, both when making a diagnosis and when deciding treatment options. Stereotyped assumptions about the race, age, gender and economic and social backgrounds of patients have all been shown to affect medical decision-making. Social prejudices have, in particular, been shown to affect diagnoses in psychiatry where there is clear evidence that assumptions about race and gender can affect diagnostic and treatment decisions (Brown, 1990; Nazroo, 2015). Some illnesses, such as coeliac disease and multiple sclerosis, are notable for the long diagnostic delays experienced by patients. It may be no accident that these are illnesses that are much more common in women (see Chapter 3). In some cases, delayed diagnosis may be because early symptoms are vague and hard to pin down. However, social stereotypes may also play a part in diagnostic delay; particularly when they result in the clinician ignoring the patient's concerns.

For some patients, a definitive diagnosis never comes. A significant minority of patients will be diagnosed as having **'medically unexplained'** symptoms. Patients with medically unexplained symptoms often have fraught relationships with health professionals. Medical literature is sometimes pejorative, treating them as a problematic group of 'heart sink' patients whose symptoms can be assumed to be psychosomatic (Stone, 2014). Treatments offered reflect this assumption, for example, cognitive behaviour therapy. A number of syndromes have been considered to be 'medically unexplained' and therefore have often been assumed to be psychological in origin. These include chronic fatigue syndrome, fibromyalgia, chronic pelvic pain and chronic back pain. The suggestion that these illnesses are psychosomatic has sometimes been controversial and disputed by patient groups. As we saw in Chapter 4, women are more likely to be diagnosed with a 'medically unexplained' condition than men. Patients without a definitive diagnosis experience heightened uncertainty, and are at particular risk of suffering blame, shame and negative labelling (Stone, 2014). Amongst this group will be some people who will eventually receive a definitive diagnosis of organic disease after years of delay. Aronowitz (2001) has suggested that as medicine has placed more emphasis on laboratory tests and less on symptoms and clinical examination, it has created new groups of 'medical orphans'. Nettleton (2021) also suggests that laboratory medicine's increased pursuit of diagnostic precision has created new groups of uncertain illnesses and thrown some groups of patients into 'diagnostic limbo'.

Contemporary diagnostic practices have clearly been successful in offering a path to effective treatment for most patients but we should not ignore the problematic experiences of some patients. Sociologists have examined the social process of diagnosis in order to identify where it can go wrong and how it can be improved. In particular, Mishler (1984) and Kleinman (1988) have considered how health professionals can be educated to become more attentive to patients narratives in order to deliver more effective and humane care. In the next section, we will look in further detail at how patients describe their experiences of illness, and what we can learn from this.

REFLECTION POINT: THE PROCESS OF DIAGNOSIS

Think about your own experiences when you last went to the doctor with a health problem:
What did you tell the doctor about why you had come? Did you just list your symptoms or did you include other reasons for visiting him/her? Did you feel the need to demonstrate that you were a 'good' patient? Did you feel you managed to say what you wanted to say?
Did the clinician listen to you? Did they interrupt you? Did you ever feel that the clinician was making judgements about you? What were you happy about in the consultation? What were you less happy with?
Does what you have just read about the sociology of diagnosis make you now look at this consultation differently? What are the lessons for you when talking to patients in your own practice?

THE MEANING OF ILLNESS

As we noted in the previous section, a number of authors have alerted us to the need to attend to patients' own stories about their illnesses and the challenges and difficulties of living with illness. Next, we will explore how people deal with the existential threats posed by illness and how people try to make sense of and account for their illness. We use stories to make sense of our world and to make life experiences more intelligible both to others and to ourselves (Greenhalgh & Calman, 2017). **Illness narratives** convey experiences of suffering through illness as well as trying to give that suffering meaning and context (Kleinman, 1988). An acute illness, such as appendicitis, may give us a sense of shock and stop normal life in its tracks, but we are likely to then get back on track as we recover. However, a long-term or potentially life-limiting illness, such as rheumatoid arthritis or cancer, may lead to more long-term disruption to our life course which we will need to come to terms with and explain.

In order to try to make sense of our experiences, we thus construct narratives about what the illness means in the context of our life and personal identity. For example, the children's author Michael Rosen gives an insightful, and often humorous, account of his own experience of severe COVID-19 and the long process of recovery (Rosen, 2022). The narratives we tell are heavily influenced by wider social expectations and cultural discourses about illness. Frank (2013) has suggested that there are a number of **'scripts'** available which offer socially acceptable ways of responding to ill health.

Frank (2013) identifies three types of **illness narrative** which each follow a particular script. The first, which he calls the **'restitution'** narrative, describes the situation where a person falls ill, seeks treatment and then recovers. This is often seen as the ideal illness narrative. It fits in with social expectations of illness. We will look at these expectations in a bit more detail in a later section when we consider the concept of the 'sick role'. For many people, however, restitution is not possible. Their illness is long term and/or life limiting. Frank describes two characteristic narratives told in relation to long term and/or life-threatening illness. The first he calls the **'quest'** narrative. Here, illness is seen as a 'journey' from which the sick person can learn self-awareness or 'personal growth'. The quest narrative underpins many published accounts of illness, since it offers a socially acceptable narrative for people with long-term illness.

The third type of narrative identified by Frank is the **'chaos'** narrative. Here, the experience of illness is dominated by uncertainty with no clear 'journey' and no clear endpoint. People whose illness is experienced as chaotic may have uncontrolled or unpredictable symptoms and/or an uncertain diagnosis or prognosis. They may also have limited support to cope with their illness or face other social pressures, such as poverty. As a result they can experience their illness as puzzling and senseless. The 'chaos' narrative reveals the sick person as vulnerable and powerless, so it is both difficult to experience and difficult for others to hear. It may be particularly difficult for health professionals to encounter as it highlights their own sense of powerlessness. There may, thus, be strong social pressures on the sick to try to account for their illness using the first two scripts identified by Frank. This creates pressures on the sick to hide their own suffering and sense of vulnerability to make others feel better. Health professionals can contribute to this pressure. Patients labelled as 'good' often follow the first two scripts while patients labelled as 'difficult' often follow the third script. Thus, well-meaning health professionals can often, unwittingly, add to the pressures on patients to hide their distress and difficulty. An example is the pressure put on cancer patients to think of their illness as a 'journey' conforming to the 'quest' narrative.

For example, Ehrenreich (2009) described being under intense pressure to look on the 'bright side' of cancer when she was diagnosed with breast cancer. Similarly, Trusson and Pilnick (2017) describe how the field of cancer care is dominated by what they call 'pink positivity'. Literature for breast cancer sufferers presents a stereotypical view of the cancer survivor, characterised by photos of smiling women in pink tracksuits taking part in a 'fun run' for a cancer charity. Celebrity accounts of living through breast cancer treatment often follow the 'restitution' narrative portraying the experience as a 'battle' from which they have emerged victorious, having learned from their experience and become better people. Patients with advanced cancer may also experience a pressure to adopt the 'quest' narrative, portraying their cancer as a heroic journey towards self-awareness. The pressure on breast cancer sufferers to show positivity can force them to censor their communication with others, making it difficult for them to express worries or discuss painful symptoms. This can result in 'survivor loneliness' among cancer survivors (Trusson & Pilnick, 2017). This discourse can also perpetuate the popular myth that positive thinking influences disease susceptibility and cancer survival. Studies have clearly demonstrated that there is no evidence to support this myth (Coyne & Tennen, 2010). This myth can burden cancer sufferers with the inference that they are to blame for the course of their illness. Trusson and Pilnick (2017) found women with breast cancer were often only able to talk honestly about their illness to other sufferers, but that some had negative experiences in patient support groups, particularly those run by health professionals which promoted 'pink positivity'. Health professionals are in a position to give patients space to honestly express their pain, distress, worries and fears, and to listen without forcing patients to conform to a socially acceptable illness narrative. Allowing patients to air their more negative feelings can help patients to deal with their distress and maintain hope. This, however, means that health professionals need to be willing to tolerate hearing the 'chaos' narrative from some patients.

> **REFLECTION POINT: ILLNESS NARRATIVES**
>
> Think about Frank's three types of illness narrative. Think of examples of the use of these three narratives from your own personal and professional experience. How helpful or unhelpful do you think Frank's typology is for understanding how we make sense of illness? In your experience, do you think that people feel under pressure to conform to a particular narrative? How helpful or unhelpful is this?

SURVIVING SERIOUS ILLNESS

Until recently, neither sociologists nor medical researchers paid much attention to the experiences of critically ill patients. Most early social research in the intensive care unit (ICU) focused on staff stress or the support of patient's families. However, as more patient narratives have emerged from people who have experienced critical care, there has been greater realisation that the subjective experiences of the critically ill are important and can affect their recovery. Patient experiences of critical illness include feelings of profound uncertainty and vulnerability; experiencing severe pain; feeling close to death; experiencing vivid and disturbing dreams and nightmares and at times feeling safe and cared for but at other times feeling helpless, alienated and afraid (Maartmann-Moe et al., 2021). There are strong parallels here with the 'chaos' narrative described by Frank (2013).

The sociologist Rier (2000) described his own experience as an ICU patient and talked about the need for patients to feel trust in staff and for staff to help patients to maintain hope. He also stressed the importance of staff making decisions in patients' best interests when they are too weak and ill to make decisions themselves. He said that his experiences challenged his strongly held beliefs in consumerism and patient choice, since he realised that he had simply been too ill to make choices. Similarly, Rosen (2022) described the value of the patient diary written for him by ICU staff, and the importance of knowing that they were willing him to get better even when he was too vulnerable and confused to do so himself. It is important that we recognise that patients who survive a stay in an ICU have been through a profound life-changing experience. To aid recovery and help them regain independence, we need to pay more attention to their subjective experiences during their illness and hospitalisation (Kean et al., 2021).

EXPERIENCING LIFE-LIMITING AND TERMINAL ILLNESS

Sociological studies of death and dying have often focused on wider social attitudes to death and dying, in particular to question whether contemporary societies 'deny' or 'hide' death (Walter, 2008). This section will focus more narrowly on what sociology can tell us about how we care for people at the end of their life.

An important early sociological study focused on communication and awareness of dying. Glaser and Strauss (2017) carried out a study of dying people in San Francisco hospitals in the 1960s. They found that, at this time, there was a common failure to disclose to patients the truth of their diagnosis and prognosis. They identified four basic patterns of communication and disclosure which they called 'awareness contexts'.

- In 'closed awareness' the patient's prognosis was not disclosed to them. A diagnosis of cancer was also sometimes withheld from patients.
- 'Suspicion awareness' occurred when the patient suspected their diagnosis but clinicians and relatives continued to withhold the truth.
- 'Mutual pretense' existed when both sides pretended to be unaware of the truth and avoided any discussion of the illness and prognosis.
- In 'open awareness' the truth was shared between patients, their families and clinicians.

Glaser and Strauss demonstrated that closed awareness led to patient isolation and poor emotional support for dying people. According to Walter (2008), their study is an example of sociological work which has positively changed healthcare practice. Recent studies have suggested that it is now normal practice to tell patients about their diagnosis and prognosis. One of the main criticisms of the work of Glaser and Strauss has been that it assumed that there was certainty about whether a patient was nearing the end of their life or not. Timmermans (1994) has suggested that some degree of uncertainty may be needed by both patients and staff to maintain hope. In reality, there may be more ambiguity and uncertainty than Glaser and Strauss allowed for. Kennedy et al., (2014) suggest that there is a need to explicitly acknowledge uncertainty when diagnosing the dying. Doctors should not overestimate their ability to determine prognosis. They suggest that where there is still some potential for recovery, however limited, decision making needs to allow for this.

Glaser and Strauss's work coincided with the development of the hospice and palliative care movement. This movement sought to provide care that allowed people to live as fully as possible until they died, by controlling distressing symptoms and providing holistic care. An important principle of hospice care, as conceived by the founder of the movement, Cicely Saunders, was to treat each patient as a unique individual who required highly personalised care. She summed up the ethos of the movement by saying:

'You matter because you are you. You matter to the last moment of your life, and we will do all we can to help you not only to die peacefully, but also to live until you die'.

(CICELY SAUNDERS INTERNATIONAL, 2021)

Since the movement was founded in the 1960s, hospices and palliative care services have been developed in many countries and have in many respects revolutionised end-of-life care. In the UK, there are now more than two hundred hospices. However, access to services has remained unequal (Oliviere et al., 2011). Seale (1995) suggested that certain groups of people were denied access to the benefits of palliative care. In particular, he believed that the elderly, particularly those in institutions, such as care homes, were least likely to receive palliative care. He called this group the 'disadvantaged dying'. Since this time, inequalities in access to palliative care have received more attention and there is more research evidence showing social inequality in the experience of dying. Pivodic et al., (2018) have corroborated Seale's suggestion that care home residents may be disadvantaged. They found that end-of-life care in care homes was variable and that a considerable proportion of care home residents died in physical and emotional distress. Corpora (2022) suggests that we take an intersectional approach to dying and argues that a 'good death' is a 'privilege' denied to many due to inequitable access to good end-of-life care. Inequalities of class, ethnicity, age, gender, sexual orientation and geographical location can all negatively affect the experience of dying and create barriers to accessing good-quality palliative care (Oliviere et al., 2011).

A study of hospice care in the NHS in the 1990s found that the 'routinization' and 'bureaucratisation' of hospice care could undermine its original ethos (James & Field, 1992). In charting the evolution of the hospice movement, Seymour (2012) noted the tendency to transform 'hospice' and 'palliative' care into a more standardised approach to 'end of life' care. This has led to recent concerns about the routinization and bureaucratisation of end-of-life care (Borgstrom & Dekker, 2022). One particular example was the introduction of the 'Liverpool Care Pathway' which attempted to introduce a standard end-of-life care pathway across the NHS. This was withdrawn after complaints by relatives that it led to poor care including the premature and forced withdrawal of nutrition, fluids and medical treatment. A review by Neuberger (2016) concluded that, despite some good care, there had been widespread misuse of the pathway due to poor training, lack of empathy and ageist attitudes among some staff. This highlighted the danger, identified by James and Field (1992), that the bureaucratisation and standardisation of palliative care can undermine its core principle of compassionate, individualised care.

REFLECTION POINT

Look back at the quotation from Cicely Saunders in this section. How do you think that health professionals can ensure a high standard of individualised, palliative care for people reaching the end of their lives in acute settings?

The Social Regulation of Illness

In this final section, we look in more detail at how society regulates and disciplines the ill and at the ways in which social reactions to illness shape the illness experience. In 1951, the American sociologist, Talcott Parsons published an account of the social role that he believed that US society expected sick people to play (Parsons, 2013).

Talcott Parsons (1902–1979) was an American sociologist and leading proponent of a branch of sociology called structural functionalism. His major works included The Social System (1951) and The Structure of Social Action (1937). Parsons was a theorist rather than an empirical researcher and developed overarching theories of the 'social system'. Structural functionalism conceives society as an integrated system in which all the parts need to work together to maintain the whole. It focuses on norms, social roles, integration, adaptation and the maintenance of social stability. Parsons made an important contribution to our understanding of societal structures. However, his work has been criticised for being socially conservative and for neglecting social inequalities and social conflict.

Parsons saw illness as disruptive to the social system, since the sick failed to perform their normal roles and obligations, such as going to work or school, or doing housework or childcare. He was influenced by the works of the psychoanalyst, Sigmund Freud, and believed people could be 'unconsciously' motivated to be ill in order to shirk their obligations. He thus thought much illness was, wholly or in part, 'psychosomatic'. Therefore, according to Parsons, illness needed to be socially regulated to maintain social 'equilibrium'. The 'sick role' thus involved a set of obligations and privileges.

According to Parsons, the sick role gave people **two rights**. Firstly, people who were sick could be exempted from their normal obligations and would be entitled to care whilst ill, and secondly, they would not be held responsible or blamed for their illness. In return for these concessions, the ill, according to Parsons, had **'two obligations'**. They must seek 'technically competent', (i.e., medical) help, and comply with treatment and they must also actively want and try to get well. Doctors were then held responsible for controlling entry to and exit from the sick role in the interests of the wider society. Doctors in return had an obligation to act in the interests of the patient and community (not out of financial self-interest); practice to a high standard of skill and knowledge and be objective and impartial in their diagnosis (Parsons, 2013).

The sick role thus conforms closely to the 'restitution' narrative of illness described by Frank (2013). This is the socially acceptable face of illness and Parsons' sick role theory was useful in highlighting the social control functions inherent in how societies manage illness. He described his theory as outlining an 'ideal type' of the sick role in the light of American cultural values (Parsons, 1979). It has thus been criticised as for its cultural narrowness, reflecting as it does, the high value placed on the work ethic and individual achievement in US society (Freund et al., 2003). It is also a very masculine view of health.

There are a number of other problems with Parsons' version of the sick role. Firstly, as we have seen in the previous section, some critically ill people are simply too ill to 'want to get well'. Secondly, and most importantly, many illnesses are not temporary. As life expectancy has increased, more people will spend significant parts of their life living with chronic illnesses, such as asthma, diabetes, arthritis or heart disease. For these people, the obligation to get well is simply not an option. Hence, there is increasing emphasis on this group's obligation to 'self-manage' their illness in order to keep fulfilling their social duties. Health services increasingly emphasise 'self-management' of long-term conditions, to minimise the demands of the long-term sick on health services and maximise their ability to stay in employment (see Chapter 7). The fact that the long-term sick may be afforded diminished rights to claim the privileges of the sick role does, however, corroborate aspects of Parsons' model (Gerhardt, 1989). We need to see his model as a description of US cultural values and attitudes towards the sick rather than as a normative prescription for the roles of sick people.

Another problem is that for some patients, as we noted in our discussion of diagnosis, access to the sick role is denied because doctors delay or fail to reach a diagnosis or make an ambiguous diagnosis, such as chronic fatigue syndrome. Parsons assumed that diagnosis was an objective and unbiased process but, as we have seen, diagnoses are socially constructed and can be affected by social biases. As we also saw when considering medicalisation and demedicalisation, diagnostic categories change over time in response to social changes. When considering diagnoses, we also saw the importance of social influences on medical judgements and the ways in which social stereotyping can enter into an individual clinician's diagnostic decisions.

Illness labels are not always welcome or positive. People do not always enter the sick role voluntarily, particularly those with mental health problems, so Parsons' assumption that people were motivated to be ill is questionable. We have already seen when we looked at help-seeking that people often delay help-seeking and treat many symptoms at home. Friends, family, employers or teachers can play an important role in sanctioning or blocking people from entering the sick role. In some cases, such as children, the elderly and the mentally ill, families or other agents may force individuals into the sick role against their will. For example, an elderly person may be forced into entering a care home because they are no longer deemed by others fit enough to live independently. Parsons' theory usefully drew attention to some widely shared cultural beliefs and assumptions about illness and his contribution highlighted the social control functions of medical institutions. People who do not conform to Parson's 'ideal type' of the sick role are often those very members of society who face stigma when they are ill because they are assumed to have broken implicit societal rules about illness (Gerhardt, 1989).

Parsons' theory drew into sharp focus the ease with which people can find themselves subject to social condemnation when sick. A number of authors have drawn attention to the moral aspects of illness. Deeply embedded social values equate good health with virtuous behaviour. In particular, illness may bring shame and blame on the chronically sick because they have failed to get well; it may bring blame on those with ambiguous diagnoses, such as fibromyalgia or myalgic encephalomyelitis (ME), because they are suspected of being malingerers who do not have a 'genuine' illness; and it may also bring blame on people with conditions, such as Type 2 diabetes, lung cancer or HIV, which the public believe to be self-inflicted. The application of blame is often neither rational nor accurate. For example, lung cancer patients reported experiencing blame for their condition even when they were lifelong non-smokers (Chapple et al., 2004). We will examine the ways in which moral evaluation of the ill can negatively affect the sick and disabled in more depth in the next chapter on long-term illness and disability.

Summary of Key Points

- There are a range of different ideas about what it means to be healthy or ill, and these have varied over time.
- Sociologists have identified a widespread process of medicalisation in contemporary society characterised by the expansion of diagnostic categories and creation of new illness labels.
- We can see diagnosis as a social process influenced by its institutional context. Perspective differences between patients and clinicians can cause poor communication, diagnostic delay and patient dissatisfaction.
- Patients make sense of their illness through 'illness narratives'. There can be pressures on patients to follow a socially acceptable 'script' when making sense of illness.
- The 'sick role' set out a socially acceptable role for the ill. It gives us insight into how societies attempt to control the sick.

Further Reading

Conrad, P., & Barker, K. (2010). The social construction of illness: Key insights and policy implications. *Journal of Health and Social Behavior, 51*(Suppl), S67–S79.

Rosen, M. (2022). *Many different kinds of love: A story of life, death and the NHS*. Penguin Books.

Trusson, D., & Pilnick, A. (2017). Between stigma and pink positivity: Women's perceptions of social interactions during and after breast cancer treatment. *Sociology of Health & Illness, 39*(3), 458–473.

References

Ahmad, W. I., & Bradby, H. (2007). Locating ethnicity and health: Exploring concepts and contexts. *Sociology of Health & Illness, 29*(6), 795–810.

Aronowitz, R. A. (2001). When do symptoms become a disease? *Annals of Internal Medicine, 134*(9 Pt 2), 803–808.

Blashfield, R. K., Keeley, J. W., Flanagan, E. H., & Miles, S. R. (2014). The cycle of classification: DSM-I through DSM-5. *Annual Review of Clinical Psychology, 10*, 25–51.

Blaxter, M. (2003). *Health and lifestyles*. Routledge.

Borgstrom, E., & Dekker, N. L. (2022). Standardising care of the dying: An ethnographic analysis of the Liverpool Care Pathway in England and the Netherlands. *Sociology of Health & Illness, 44*(9), 1445–1460.

Brown, P. (1990). The name game: Toward a sociology of diagnosis. *The Journal of Mind and Behavior, 11*, 385–406.

Calnan, M. (1987). *Health and illness: The lay perspective*. Tavistock Publications.

Chapple, A., Ziebland, S., & McPherson, A. (2004). Stigma, shame, and blame experienced by patients with lung cancer: Qualitative study. *BMJ, 328*(7454), 1470.

Cicely Saunders International. (2021). *You matter because you are you: An action plan for better palliative care*. Retrieved January 13, 2024, from. https://csiweb.pos-pal.co.uk/csi-content/uploads/2021/01/Cicely-Saunders-Manifesto-A4-multipage_Jan2021-2.pdf.

Conrad, P., & Barker, K. K. (2010). The social construction of illness: Key insights and policy implications. *Journal of Health and Social Behavior, 51*(Suppl), S67–S79.

Conrad, P., & Leiter, V. (2004). Medicalization, markets and consumers. *Journal of Health and Social Behavior*, 158–176.

Cornford, C. S., & Cornford, H. M. (1999). 'I'm only here because of my family': A study of lay referral networks. *The British Journal of General Practice, 49*(445), 617.

Corpora, M. (2022). The privilege of a good death: An intersectional perspective on dying a good death in America. *The Gerontologist, 62*(5), 773–779.

Coyle, J. (1999). Exploring the meaning of 'dissatisfaction' with health care: The importance of 'personal identity threat. *Sociology of Health & Illness, 21*(1), 95–123.

Coyne, J. C., & Tennen, H. (2010). Positive psychology in cancer care: Bad science, exaggerated claims, and unproven medicine. *Annals of Behavioral Medicine, 39*(1), 16–26.

Crawford, R. (1980). Healthism and the medicalization of everyday life. *International Journal of Health Services, 10*(3), 365–388.

Dickinson, T., Cook, M., Playle, J., & Hallett, C. (2012). Queer 'treatments': Giving a voice to former patients who received treatments for their 'sexual deviations.' *Journal of Clinical Nursing, 21*(9–10), 1345–1354.

Ebeling, M. (2011). Get with the Program!: Pharmaceutical marketing, symptom checklists and self-diagnosis. *Social Science & Medicine, 73*(6), 825–832.

Ehrenreich, B. (2009). *Smile or die: How positive thinking fooled America and the world.* Granta Books.

Frank, A. W. (2013). *The wounded storyteller: Body, illness, and ethics.* University of Chicago Press.

Freidson, E. (1970). *Profession of medicine.* Dodds Mead.

Freund, P. E. S., McGuire, M. B., & Podhurst, L. S. (2003). *Health, illness, and the social body: A critical sociology.* Prentice Hall.

Gerhardt, U. (1989). *Ideas about illness: An intellectual and political history of medical sociology.* Macmillan Ltd.

Glaser, B. G., & Strauss, A. L. (2017). *Awareness of dying.* Routledge.

Greenhalgh, T., & Calman, K. (2017). *What seems to be the trouble? Stories in illness and healthcare.* CRC Press.

Illich, I. (1975). *Medical nemesis: The expropriation of health.* Calder & Boyars.

James, N., & Field, D. (1992). The routinization of hospice: Charisma and bureaucratization. *Social Science & Medicine, 34*(12), 1363–1375.

Jewson, N. D. (1976). The disappearance of the sick-man from medical cosmology, 1770–1870. *Sociology, 10*(2), 225–244.

Jutel, A. (2009). Sociology of diagnosis: A preliminary review. *Sociology of Health & Illness, 31*(2), 278–299.

Kean, S., Donaghy, E., Bancroft, A., Clegg, G., & Rodgers, S. (2021). Theorising survivorship after intensive care: A systematic review of patient and family experiences. *Journal of Clinical Nursing, 30*(17–18), 2584–2610.

Kennedy, C., Brooks-Young, P., Gray, C. B., Larkin, P., Connolly, M., Wilde-Larsson, B., & Chater, S. (2014). Diagnosing dying: An integrative literature review. *BMJ Supportive & Palliative Care, 4*, 263–270.

Kleinman, A. (1988). *The illness narratives: Suffering, healing and the human condition.* Basic Books.

Maartmann-Moe, C. C., Solberg, M. T., Larsen, M. H., & Steindal, S. A. (2021). Patients' memories from intensive care unit: A qualitative systematic review. *Nursing Open, 8*(5), 2221–2234.

Macintyre, S., McKay, L., & Ellaway, A. (2006). Lay concepts of the relative importance of different influences on health; are there major socio-demographic variations? *Health Education Research, 21*(5), 731–739.

Malterud, K., & Thesen, J. (2008). When the helper humiliates the patient: A qualitative study about unintended intimidations. *Scandinavian Journal of Public Health, 36*(1), 92–98.

Malterud, K. (2005). Humiliation instead of care? *The Lancet, 366*(9488), 785–786.

Mishler, E. G. (1984). *The discourse of medicine: Dialectics of medical interviews.* Ablex Publishing Corp.

Morgan, M., & Thomas, M. (2009). Lay and professional constructions of time: Implications for illness behaviour and management of a chronic condition. *Sociology, 43*(3), 555–572.

Moynihan, R., Doust, J., & Henry, D. (2012). Preventing overdiagnosis: How to stop harming the healthy. *BMJ, 344*, e3502.

Moynihan, R., Heath, I., & Henry, D. (2002). Selling sickness: The pharmaceutical industry and disease mongering commentary: Medicalisation of risk factors. *BMJ, 324*(7342), 886–891.

Navarro, V. (1975). The industrialization of fetishism or the fetishism of industrialization: A critique of Ivan Illich. *Social Science & Medicine, 9*(7), 351–363.

Nazroo, J. Y. (2015). Ethnic inequalities in severe mental disorders: Where is the harm? *Social Psychiatry and Psychiatric Epidemiology, 50*(7), 1065–1067.

Nettleton, S. (2021). *The sociology of health and illness.* Polity Press.

Nettleton, S., Burrows, R., & O'Malley, L. (2005). The mundane realities of the everyday lay use of the internet for health, and their consequences for media convergence. *Sociology of Health & Illness, 27*(7), 972–992.

Neuberger, J. (2016). The Liverpool Care Pathway: What went right and what went wrong. *British Journal of Hospital Medicine, 77*(3), 172–174.

Oliviere, D., Monroe, B., & Payne, S. (Eds.). (2011). *Death, dying, and social differences.* Oxford University Press.

Parsons, T. (1979). Definitions of health and illness in light of American values and social structure. In E. Jaco (Ed.), *Patients, physicians and illness* (pp. 120–144). Collier Macmillan: The Free Press.

Parsons, T. (2013). *The social system*. Routledge.

Pivodic, L., Smets, T., Van den Noortgate, N., Onwuteaka-Philipsen, B. D., Engels, Y., Szczerbińska, K., & Van den Block, L. (2018). Quality of dying and quality of end-of-life care of nursing home residents in six countries: An epidemiological study. *Palliative Medicine, 32*(10), 1584–1595.

Rier, D. (2000). The missing voice of the critically ill: A medical sociologist's first-person account. *Sociology of Health & Illness, 22*(1), 68–93.

Rosen, M. (2022). *Many different kinds of love: A story of life death and the NHS*. Penguin Books.

Scott, S. (2006). The medicalisation of shyness: From social misfits to social fitness. *Sociology of Health & Illness, 28*(2), 133–153.

Seale, C. (1995). Heroic death. *Sociology, 29*(4), 597–613.

Seymour, J. (2012). Looking back, looking forward: The evolution of palliative and end-of-life care in England. *Mortality, 17*(1), 1–17.

Sloan, M., Harwood, R., Sutton, S., D'Cruz, D., Howard, P., Wincup, C., Brimicombe, J., & Gordon, C. (2020). Medically explained symptoms: A mixed methods study of diagnostic, symptom and support experiences of patients with lupus and related systemic autoimmune diseases. *Rheumatology advances in practice, 4*(1), 1–11.

Smith, L. K., Pope, C., & Botha, J. L. (2005). Patients' help-seeking experiences and delay in cancer presentation: A qualitative synthesis. *The Lancet, 366*(9488), 825–831.

Stone, L. (2014). Blame, shame and hopelessness: Medically unexplained symptoms and the 'heartsink' experience. *Australian Family Physician, 43*(4), 191–195.

Timmermans, S. (1994). Dying of awareness: The theory of awareness contexts revisited. *Sociology of Health & Illness, 16*(3), 322–339.

Trusson, D., & Pilnick, A. (2017). Between stigma and pink positivity: Women's perceptions of social interactions during and after breast cancer treatment. *Sociology of Health & Illness, 39*(3), 458–473.

Walter, T. (2008). The sociology of death. *Sociology Compass, 2*(1), 317–336.

WHO. (1946). *Constitution of the World Health Organisation*. Retrieved January 9, 2024, from. https://www.who.int/about/accountability/governance/constitution.

Zola, I. K. (1972). Medicine as an institution of social control. *The Sociological Review, 20*(4), 487–504.

Zola, I. K. (1973). Pathways to the doctor—From person to patient. Social Science & Medicine, 7(9), 677–689.

Living With Long-Term Illness and Disability

The first part of this chapter will consider what it is like to live with a long-term illness that affects daily life. It will discuss sociological research into how long-term illness has affected people's lives, sense of self and social identity. The 'symbolic interactionist' perspective which informs these studies will be introduced. The chapter will then examine policy and practice which encourages self-management of long-term illness and question whether or not this is empowering for patients. It will also discuss stereotyping, labelling and stigma and their adverse effects on people with long-term illness and disability.

The second part of this chapter will look more specifically at disability and consider the contribution that the disabled rights movement has made to our understanding of disability. It will also discuss the ways in which disability activists have challenged orthodox medical and sociological approaches to long-term illness and disability. It will look at the social model of disability and contrast this with the biomedical model. It will consider the importance of overcoming disabling barriers to social participation and the need to provide the long-term sick and disabled with both social rights and control over the social and medical support that they receive.

Living With Long-Term Illness

CHANGING PATTERNS OF LONG-TERM ILLNESS

Since the nineteenth century, many affluent industrial societies have seen an increase in life expectancy due to a reduction in early deaths from infectious diseases. As a result, life expectancy has increased, but so has the prevalence of long-term illness. This is due to an ageing population, but also, to a lesser extent, to the survival of children and young people with illnesses and disabilities who would previously have died in infancy. We should see this increased survival as good news. However, as longevity has increased, politicians, economists and policymakers have started to worry about the 'burden' of the old, disabled and long-term sick. Dorling (2011) has challenged these assumptions arguing that older people and people with disabilities can still be useful and productive members of society. He says that their marginalisation is largely due to social discrimination and inequalities. These exacerbate their problems and diminish their ability to contribute to society.

There is, however, no doubt that long-term illness and disability are considerable challenges to societies, healthcare systems and, most importantly, the people who suffer from them. In the UK, average life expectancy was 81 in 2019 while average healthy life expectancy is lower, at around 64 years, although this is unequally distributed (see Chapter 2). Thus, many people spend a considerable part of their life living with one or more long-term conditions.

Long-term conditions have traditionally been neglected by healthcare systems just as are older people. Working with people with long-term illness and disability can be an unpopular area of medicine, as it challenges the identities of doctors as people who cure people. Working with older people is also devalued due to ageist attitudes. Thus, specialties dealing with long-term disabling conditions, such as rheumatology, can be the least popular and lowest-funded areas of medicine, traditionally described as 'Cinderella specialties' (Bennett et al., 1972). Although long-term conditions are most prevalent in people over 60, there are also large numbers of younger people affected, with 14% of people under 40 suffering from a long-term condition (Kings Fund, 2013). Among the most common long-term illnesses in the UK are asthma, diabetes, chronic obstructive pulmonary disease (COPD), arthritis, heart disease and depression. The societal challenge is to help people with long-term conditions and disabilities to continue to live happy and successful lives.

Inequalities and Long-Term Illness

Long-term conditions are far more prevalent in older people, but their prevalence is also affected by inequalities of class, race, gender and geographical location. Prevalence is particularly high in inner cities where rates of both physical and mental ill health are high and strongly linked to deprivation (Hatch et al., 2011). People living in the most deprived fifth of geographical areas had, on average, two or more long-term conditions by the age of 61 (see also Chapter 2). By contrast, people in the least deprived areas can expect to live an extra 10 years free of long-term illness (Bibby et al., 2020).

There are also marked disparities in healthy life expectancy between ethnic groups. Over half of people from ethnic minorities have a lower than average healthy life expectancy, and this is likely to be largely due to the intersection of ethnicity and socioeconomic inequalities (Hayanga et al., 2022; Wohland et al., 2015).

Gender inequalities in the prevalence of long-term conditions also exist; women can expect to live for a shorter time in good health than men. We saw in Chapter 3 that long-term conditions suffered by women are often taken less seriously than conditions suffered mainly by men (Malmusi et al., 2012). Women carry a higher burden of morbidity earlier in life, and this can be explained by factors linked to gender inequalities such as inequalities in the workplace, the increased burden of unpaid work carried by women within the family and, in some instances, poorer care (Borrell et al., 2014).

THE EXPERIENCE OF LONG-TERM ILLNESS

Interactionist Approaches to the Experience of Illness

Much of the work that has been carried out on the experience of illness has been conducted using the **'symbolic interactionist'** perspective. Studies drawing on this approach often use in-depth interviews to understand how people view and experience their world. Interactionist research can also involve observations of social situations, such as doctor–patient consultations, since interactionists believe that our understanding of the world is shaped through our interactions with others.

Symbolic interactionism was founded by the US social scientist George Herbert Mead (1862–1931). He highlighted the unique nature of human consciousness arguing that humans were distinctive in being capable of internal reflection. He said people communicate through shared symbols, especially through language, and that the human world is built on the meanings people attach to these symbols. For example, health professionals' uniforms convey symbolic meanings.

Mead believed that people develop a sense of self through interaction with others and this process involves internalising the symbolic meanings conveyed to them by others. He said that the process of developing a sense of self begins with childhood socialisation. Through socialisation people develop subjective beliefs about the expectations others have of them and they try to respond to these expectations.

Blumer (1986) said symbolic interactionism had three key ideas. Firstly, action is based on meaning. Secondly, people develop an understanding of the meaning of things through interaction. Thirdly, people make sense of the meaning of interaction through internal reflection.

For interactionists, the key to understanding how people deal with illness is to understand what illness means to them. Interactionists focus on the social world at a 'micro' level. For example, they may examine face-to-face interactions to look at how people build an understanding of the meaning of their illness through their interactions with others. Interactionists see the making of meaning as a dynamic process. For example, we saw in the last chapter how people understood the meaning of their symptoms and made decisions about help-seeking through interaction with other people. Interactionists believe that society is built from these everyday interactions. Thus, interactionists focus on social actions and interactions at a micro level rather than on wider societal structures or social institutions.

Interactionists believe that how we deal with and make sense of an experience, such as diagnosis with a long-term illness, will be shaped by others around us, such as family, friends, work colleagues and health professionals. The interactionist approach has proved popular not only with medical sociologists but also with health professionals, such as nurses who want to understand how people experience illness (Tower et al., 2012).

There have been some criticisms of the limitations of interactionism. Its focus on 'micro'-level interaction means it can tend to ignore structural issues, such as inequality. We will see this later when we examine stigma. We will look at some of its findings about long-term illness next.

Disruption to Everyday Life

Long-term illness can disrupt people's lives in many ways. In an early study, Bury (1982) described illness as causing **'biographical disruption'**. Building on this work, Williams (2001) suggests it disrupts our 'taken for granted assumptions' and 'structures of everyday life' (p. 43), that is, our assumptions about our everyday world and its routines. For example, an illness, such as inflammatory bowel disease (IBD), entails regular illness episodes involving disabling symptoms, such as pain, bleeding, fatigue and diarrhoea. Such illnesses can suddenly throw our everyday life into disarray, threatening our ability to engage in activities that we once took for granted (Saunders, 2017). Saunders found that young people with IBD experienced their life as 'going round in circles'. They experienced periods of remission that enabled them to get their life back on track only to find it knocked off course again by another episode of illness.

People with mental health problems can also experience biographical disruption, through the emotional pain of an illness, such as depression (Apesoa-Varano, 2015). Long-term illness can mean people may not know from day to day whether they are going to feel well enough to attend a social event. go to work, take a planned holiday etc. They may find it even harder to make longer-term plans, such as going to university, finding a new job, getting married, buying a house or having children.

Williams (2001) says that long-term illnesses can also disrupt our 'explanatory frameworks'. Firstly, they raise questions, such as 'why me?' which can be confusing, hard to answer and undermining to our sense of self. We have seen that we form our sense of self through interactions with others. Thus, we will have already internalised a set of symbolic ideas and beliefs about the meaning of illness and the status of sick people prior to becoming ill ourselves. As a result, illness is disruptive not only because of its practical consequences but also because of what it symbolises and how this threatens our sense of self. Illness can often have very negative cultural connotations and these can make us feel like a lesser person. According to Charmaz (1983), long-term illness can lead people to feel that their carefully constructed self-image is 'crumbling away' in the face of illness. Long-term illnesses, such as cancer, heart disease or multiple sclerosis that are 'life limiting' may be even more threatening to our sense of self. They starkly face us with a threat to our very existence, even if we are able to live with them for many years.

Uncertainty

One factor which makes a large contribution to the disruptive impact of long-term illness is its **uncertainty**. People with long-term illness may have already experienced a long period of **diagnostic uncertainty** before receiving a diagnosis and a clear explanation for their symptoms. Diagnosis can, at first, come as a relief from uncertainty but this may quickly give way to uncertainty about how the diagnosis is going to affect their day-to-day life and future. For example, day-to-day life may be affected by **symptom uncertainty** and this is particularly true of illnesses characterised by fluctuating symptoms, such as rheumatoid arthritis (RA) and IBD. People with RA may feel well enough to plan an activity one day but the next day wake up to pain, fatigue and restricted mobility. Day-to-day life can, therefore, become extremely difficult to plan. People may also experience **'prognostic uncertainty'**. Will their illness follow a stable course or will they experience a steep and rapid decline in health leading to death?

We call the course of illness; an **'illness trajectory'**. The shape of an illness trajectory varies across different illnesses. Corbin and Strauss have suggested a number of different possible phases to illness trajectories (Corbin & Strauss, 1991; Corbin, 1998). Phases in an illness trajectory can include periods of stability, where symptoms are well controlled so that something resembling normal life is possible, interspersed with periods of instability when symptoms flare up. Instability can then lead to acute illness or an illness crisis involving hospitalisation. For example, a person with asthma may experience a long period of stability with symptoms under good control punctuated with acute exacerbations of illness requiring emergency treatment. A life-limiting illness, such as heart failure, may involve a long period of stability when the illness is well controlled, but this will eventually give way to instability and/or periods of crisis. This can then lead to a downward phase involving slow or rapid decline and eventual death. Understanding illness trajectories can help both patients and health professionals to intervene to control unstable periods of illness before crises develop or deterioration occurs.

Illness as Work

Living with a long-term illness is very hard work and managing the illness and its effects is often very time-consuming. Corbin and Strauss (1985) have suggested that people living with long-term illness engage in several types of work in order to manage their illness. Firstly, **'illness work'** involves dealing with health professionals; monitoring and managing symptoms; following treatment plans; carrying out diagnostic tests and preventing and managing acute episodes of illness. Jowsey and Yen (2012) suggest that some chronically ill people can spend two hours per day or more on such activities, limiting their time for normal life. Secondly, they need to carry out **'everyday life work'**, such as paid work, managing the home meals and child care and have to adapt this work to manage it whilst ill or disabled. Corbin and Strauss suggest that the ill also have to carry out what they call **'sentimental work'**. This involves managing their own and other people's emotions. This can be particularly difficult if people's reactions are negative or stigmatising.

Finally, people carry out **'biographical work'** to deal with the impact of the illness on their life course and biography. In other words, they try to manage and mitigate biographical disruption.

Thus, the uncertainties of being diagnosed with a long-term illness can force people to rethink their life plans. For some, this can be a profoundly painful process of giving up their hopes and dreams for the future. People often have to re-think their life story to incorporate an explanation of the onset and progress of their illness and its impact on their life course. Williams (1984) called this process **'narrative reconstruction'**. Long-term illness can force people to reappraise all their normal routines and future life plans with profound implications for their sense of self. In summary, people with long-term illness have to devise a large number of practical, cognitive and emotional adjustments in order to carry on with everyday life successfully.

Biographical Reconstruction and Inequalities

Bury (1982) suggested that adjustment to long-term illness involved **'biographical reconstruction'** through which people mobilise resources to help them deal with their changed status. The ability to mobilise these resources is affected by social inequalities. Not only are people from less affluent backgrounds more likely to contract long-term illnesses; they also have less access to the resources that may reduce the disruption that the illness may cause to their lives. Long-term illness often has serious financial consequences leading to loss of employment income as well as additional costs imposed by the illness itself. These can involve treatment costs as well as increases in everyday costs, such as extra heating and travel costs. For the less well-off, long-term illness and disability may be compounded by poverty. By contrast, the more affluent may be able to afford to pay for aids and adaptations as well as people to help with those tasks that they can no longer do themselves, thereby retaining more control over their lives.

The affluent may also have more control over their environment and easier access to a supportive social network (Tausig, 2013). This includes not only the immediate family and household but the wider neighbourhood and community. The more affluent usually live in neighbourhoods with better facilities and services. They also have the cultural resources (or 'cultural capital') to enable them to interact more assertively with health care institutions in order to get their needs met (Potter et al., 2018).

A variety of social and material resources can help people to rebuild a meaningful life with a long-term illness, whereas a lack of such resources can mean the path of someone with a long-term illness can be strewn with insurmountable obstacles (Bury, 1982). For example, the person with a respiratory illness who is a tenant living in substandard housing may have no power to manage the environmental conditions which exacerbate their illness (Collins, 2005). A lack of supportive resources can thus impair both coping and biographical reconstruction, potentially leading to the loss of a sense of self and social isolation. The long-term sick and disabled may also be more likely to experience disrupted roles and relationships in those social contexts in which people with long-term illness or disability are socially excluded and stigmatised. Similarly, they will experience disruption to their careers more often in workplaces that are reluctant to make accommodations for people with impairments.

Dealing With Health Services

We have said that living with long-term illness is hard work and will now consider one aspect of this in more detail. As Jowsey and Yen (2012) have noted, the **'illness work'** associated with long-term illness can be time-consuming. Furthermore, when this also involves encounters with health professionals and visits to hospitals, clinics etc., the long-term sick will quickly learn that these institutions operate to their own timetables which take little account of the difficulties these may cause to their patients. Illnesses often have their own particular timetables or rhythms. The person with rheumatoid arthritis, for example, may need to make time to get up slowly in order to get over morning joint stiffness, but clinic timetables rarely take into account these health-related needs. It is often interactions with healthcare institutions that are the most time-consuming and stressful aspects of illness management for the long-term sick. These can typically involve long waits in clinics, multiple tests on different days and times and long travel times. As services have become more fragmented, for many patients, it can also mean retelling the story of their illness to a dizzying array of different health professionals. This is exacerbated for people with more than one long-term condition who can find that a lack of care coordination means they are travelling long distances to several different hospitals and/or clinics and dealing with many different staff (Cowie et al., 2009). For these people, being ill can come to feel like a full-time job. Yet, there is rarely much appreciation of these difficulties on the part of healthcare institutions (Jowsey et al., 2016).

Self-Management of Long-Term Illness

A key objective of contemporary health policy and practice relating to long-term illness has been to enforce the expectation that patients will **'self-manage'** their condition at home. For the patient, this entails a sharp increase in **'illness work'**. A basic example might be an asthma patient who is expected to monitor their condition at home using a peak flow meter and pulse oximeter and to adjust their medication according to the readings taken. The idea of self-management in long-term illness first gained prominence in the 1990s and was based on work with arthritis patients in the US. Lorig and Holman (2003) developed a series of self-management training programmes based on psychological theories of 'self-efficacy'. They suggested that the patient should be trained to take responsibility for a range of management tasks including 'problem solving', 'resource utilisation' and lifelong 'self-monitoring and self-evaluation' (McCorkle et al., 2011). This is a managerialist approach to illness (see Chapter 9). Thus, the long-term sick were being asked to become project managers, with the management of their illness assigned as their lifelong project of work.

Lorig and Holman (2003) argued that their programmes could help patients to minimise their symptoms and gain more control over their condition. They also argued that self-management would 'empower' patients. Their ideas were picked up by policymakers in a number of countries looking for ways to reduce healthcare costs. Self-management, it was argued, could provide a low-cost way for patients to manage their illness at home, thus reducing their use of acute services, particularly emergency care. This, it was argued, could cut healthcare costs and facilitate a reduction in in-patient beds. In the UK, a Department of Health (DOH) report envisaged a three-tier pyramid of NHS care with professional care at the top for the sickest, high-risk patients, 'shared care' for those in the middle and the majority of patients at the bottom of the pyramid being expected to manage their illness themselves (DOH, 2004). It was argued by some health service managers that the NHS needed to encourage the 'flat-pack patient' who was prepared to shoulder more of the work and costs of care themselves (rather like the IKEA customer who is expected to build their own bookshelves) (Cayton, 2006). In other words, self-management involved 'cost-shifting' from health services to patients (see McDonaldization in Chapter 9). In the UK, the 'Expert Patient' programme was introduced to train patients in self-management. This was promoted by the chief medical officer of the English NHS with the claim that self-management would improve patient outcomes, life expectancy and quality of life and create a new era of 'optimism and opportunity' (Donaldson, 2003).

Subsequent evaluations of self-management programmes have shown that the claims made for them were greatly overstated. While programme outcomes have shown some improvements in psychological variables, such as self-efficacy, they have had only minor impacts on disease outcomes with often small improvements noted in only a few conditions, such as asthma and diabetes. There has also been little evidence that they have reduced use of services or healthcare costs (Greenhalgh, 2009). The evidence has also suggested that, while some patients find them beneficial and empowering, their effects may be short term. Furthermore, they may only be most suitable for selected patients who have enough resources to benefit from them (Newbould et al., 2006).

Self-management programmes focus on psychological 'adjustment' to illness. They are thus individualistic in nature and blind both to the social context within which the individual has to try to manage their illness, or the tools available to them. Patients, however, have to manage their illness within the realities of their social situation and some patients will have limited opportunities to control factors that negatively affect their illness, such as poor work conditions. People with long-term illness may also have many other demands on them. For example, they may be shouldering heavy caring responsibilities, such as caring for a spouse with dementia. They may have an employer who is unwilling to make adjustments to help them manage their condition. Hinder and Greenhalgh (2012) suggest that a lack of engagement with self-management can be an understandable response to stretched capacity and resources. This is where the self-management model (like the IKEA bookcase) can fall down.

Greenhalgh (2009) suggests that we need a more holistic model for managing long-term illness which takes a person's social context much more into account. Nevertheless, the expectations that patients with long-term illness will self-manage their condition have steadily increased. As we will see in Chapter 10, inpatient beds in the NHS have declined sharply over the last 20 years, putting more pressure on community services (Griffin, 2022). Health professionals' expectations that patients will self-manage long-term illnesses were further accelerated by the COVID-19 pandemic which severely restricted access to face-to-face care. There is evidence that this situation worsened outcomes and quality of life for some patients (Miller et al., 2020). This suggests that rather than being 'empowering', self-management is often imposed and is being employed as a form of care rationing. Health professionals have also been found to label patients according to their compliance with self-management. For example, McDonald et al. (2008) found that community nurses labelled patients as 'good' or 'bad' self-managers depending on their commitment to self-management regimes, with little consideration of the circumstances within which people were trying to manage their illness. We will pick up the issue of labelling and moral evaluation of patients in the next section.

REFLECTION POINT

There is increased emphasis on the patient self-managing their long-term illness in contemporary healthcare. How do you think this positively impacts on patients? How do you think this negatively impacts on patients?

EXPERIENCING STIGMA, DISCRIMINATION AND SOCIAL EXCLUSION

Labelling

A case study by Williams (2002) of a rheumatology patient found that she, in common with other people with long-term illness, struggled to maintain self-respect in the face of a variety of negative ideas about the sick; namely, that the sick and disabled were an encumbrance and a burden on society; that sickness was associated with uncleanliness and that the sick were indebted to others and to society. Williams associated this with deep rooted, cultural ideas which value individualism and the work ethic while blaming the victims of ill health for their own suffering. Williams said that these cultural ideas have led to negative moral evaluations of the sick. We can see this in the negative public discourse about people on disability benefits. Charmaz (2020) argues that recent public policy and political discourse have added to the stigmatisation of the disabled and chronically sick. This can lead to pejorative labels being attached to those who are sick, even when their ill health has occurred through no fault of their own, as was the case for the rheumatoid arthritis patient studied by Williams (2002). This can lead to a process of labelling which sets those who are sick apart from 'normal' people.

Labelling is the social process whereby people are given a negative label that marks them out as different from the 'normal' population. It was first described by Howard Becker in 1963 (Becker, 2008, 2018). Labelling can occur when people are given a medical diagnosis, particularly if that label is seen by others to override other aspects of their identity. When this occurs, we call this new identity a **'master status'** (Becker, 2008). For example, we might come to view someone primarily as mentally ill, disabled or a cancer patient and allow this to override, in our minds, all other aspects of their identity, such as that of nurse, teacher or parent. These labels, once attached, can have lasting consequences. We come to associate the person with the cultural stereotypes which we associate with that particular label and we start to make assumptions about them. This may change the way we think about them and talk to them.

People who have been labelled can feel forced to comply with the societal expectations and stereotypes applied to people with that label. They find themselves trapped by the label. For example, school children with disabilities frequently find themselves socially excluded or forced into the company of other disabled children with whom they may have little in common apart from the fact that they are disabled (Davis & Watson, 2001). This can reinforce their identification with the label of 'disabled child'. Labelling may lead to people finding that their options are increasingly closed off, so that they are forced into the role expected of people with their label. For example, a classic study first published in the 1960s showed that there are certain stereotyped expectations of blind people to which a person who has lost their sight may be expected to conform (Scott, 2017). Thus, the process of labelling can constrain people's life chances, in many ways, limiting their career options and social life.

Health Professionals' Labelling of Patients

Studies over the last 50 years have shown that health professionals make moral judgements about patients and may classify them as 'good', 'bad', 'difficult', 'popular' or 'unpopular'. A classic early study also indicated that the negative labelling of patients can lead to worse care with health professionals less willing to engage with 'unpopular' patients (Stockwell, 1972). Johnson and Webb (1995) suggested that nurses make 'social judgements' about patients and that the most frequent negative label was that patients were 'demanding'. Labels attributed by health professionals can, in part, reflect wider social attitudes towards particular groups. Thus, patients with mental health problems, such as drug users, can be stigmatised in acute settings. This can lead to patients with mental health problems being ignored, avoided or treated in a coercive and/or judgemental manner (Perry et al., 2020). Cresswell (2020) found similar negative moral evaluations of people who self-harm by emergency department (ED) staff. This prejudice is not unique to acute settings however. Griffiths (2001), for example, found that community mental health teams also used negative moral evaluations of their patients to justify delaying access to care.

In an early study of emergency department staff, Jeffery (1979) suggested that staff distinguished 'good' patients from 'rubbish'. 'Rubbish' included 'drunks', 'trivia' and 'tramps'. Jeffery argued that 'rubbish' broke the unwritten rules of the emergency department which were that patients should not be responsible for their illness; their illness should warrant emergency treatment and they should cooperate with staff. Jeffery argued that staff punished 'rubbish' through longer waits and unsympathetic treatment. Later studies showed negative labels applied to patients for similar reasons though seldom expressed in such unguarded language (Strudwick, 2016). This kind of labelling reinforces a 'moral order' in which certain types of patient are seen as 'good' or 'proper' to the setting while others are seen as illegitimate, often by being labelled as 'social' rather than 'medical' problems. Ageism can also contribute to negative labelling of patients and age discrimination in healthcare has been described as a pervasive problem (Nemiroff, 2022). Those subject to negative labelling are often older people with long-term illnesses who are judged by health professionals to have a limited medical future (Latimer, 1997). It is these patients who may all too frequently find themselves relabelled as 'inappropriate attenders', 'frequent flyers' or 'bed blockers' (see Chapter 10). The existence of negative labelling of patients within healthcare can both perpetuate bias and damage care standards (Valdez, 2021). We call this type of negative labelling **'stigma'** and will now explore this concept in more detail.

REFLECTION POINT

Think of examples of negative labelling of patients that you have encountered. What types of patients were negatively labelled? Why do you think this process of labelling occurred? What do you think the consequences of labelling were for the patient? How do you think that patient labelling might be discouraged in healthcare settings?

Stigma

We introduced the concept of **stigma** in Chapter 1 in relation to poverty stigma and in Chapter 5 in relation to fat shaming and weight stigma. Goffman (2009) described stigma as involving a particular type of negative labelling. He said that stigmatising labels are applied to people who have an 'attribute' that is perceived as 'deeply discrediting' in the eyes of a particular society or group. Attributes that are seen as discrediting might include bodily differences, such as facial disfigurement or disability. Goffman says that discredited attributes can also include presumed 'character flaws', such as being unemployed, having a criminal record or a history of mental illness. The application of a stigmatising label may not be objective, fair or true but it is real in its consequences for the individual facing stigma.

Erving Goffman (1922–1982) was a Canadian sociologist. He was seen as a leading figure in interactionist sociology although he did not identify himself as a symbolic interactionist. Goffman studied how people make sense of their world in everyday life through their interactions with others. He used a 'dramaturgical' perspective likening social life to a drama in which individuals have to draw on pre-existing scripts and props and carefully manage 'front stage' and 'back stage' areas of their environment to interact successfully in social situations. Of particular interest to health professionals are, firstly, his book 'Stigma: Notes on the Management of Spoiled Identity', published in 1963, and, secondly, his ethnographic study of a psychiatric hospital; 'Asylums: Essays on the Social Situation of Mental Patients and Other Inmates', published in 1961. This book played an important role in the reform of psychiatric institutions in the late twentieth century. Although Goffman worked within the tradition of symbolic interactionism there were some important differences between his work and that of other interactionist sociologists, particularly in his analysis of institutions. He used the concept of the 'interaction order' to illuminate the fixed and ritualised nature of much social interaction and the ways in which this led to the persistence of institutionalised regimes.

A stigmatising label discredits an individual to the extent that they are no longer seen as a 'usual person'. Instead, according to Goffman, stigma 'spoils' their identity and redefines them as a 'tainted' and 'discredited' person. Goffman distinguished two different situations facing people who are stigmatised. In the first case, the stigmatised attribute is visible and impossible to hide. Examples could include a person with facial disfigurement or someone with cerebral palsy. Goffman describes this group of people as **'discredited'**. They may face **'enacted stigma'** in every social situation. Their dilemmas involve deciding what techniques to use to manage other people's negative reactions to them; whether these involve avoidance, curious stares, patronising looks of pity or outright hostility and abuse. They may try a variety of tactics to manage other people's difficult behaviours, such as reacting with humour, ignoring them or confronting them head-on. They may also try to 'cover' the most obvious signs of their disability, even if they cannot hide it completely. In doing so, they are trying to be less conspicuous in the hope that this might minimise the negative reactions of other people. Dealing with these situations on a day-to-day basis can be hard work and exhausting.

In the second situation, people have a 'discrediting' attribute that can be concealed. In this case Goffman says they are **'discreditable'**, since, if the attribute is disclosed, they may face stigma and labelling but they have some scope for hiding it. This might apply to someone with a largely invisible illness, such as the person who has epilepsy, is HIV positive or has a history of mental illness. In this case, the person can **'pass'** as 'normal' in most social situations. The dilemmas for this group of people are twofold. Firstly, in order to 'pass' they may need to conceal the discrediting attribute, for example by wearing a prosthesis and adapted clothing to conceal a limb amputation. Depending on the type of problem involved, concealment can involve varying amounts of work and can sometimes interfere with treatment. An example would be an asthma sufferer who does not want to be seen using an inhaler at work.

Secondly, the 'discreditable' will face dilemmas about how to manage their personal information. Who should they tell and when and how should they reveal potentially discrediting information? For example, should they tell people they have had cancer? Do they need to tell their employer about their medical history? This group of people may feel considerable anxiety about revealing information about themselves, and the reactions they may face from other people.

Examples: Experiencing 'Discredited' and 'Discreditable' Stigma

I say 'Well, I've not been so good, I've been having treatment'. 'For what?' 'Cancer'. Step back in amazement and shock! That sort of thing… I know that it's a bit like saying 'I've just gone down with leprosy' or something. And they think, well, if they get too near they might catch it. Some people are too sensitive to delve into it, the fact you've been, you've told them you have cancer is enough and they recoil, recoil. They say 'Poor old Tom, he's got cancer and he'll not make Christmas'.

(THOMAS, 2010, p. 51)

You know how kids are, they like everything to be the same, like everybody should be the same.… I was the only disabled student in a student body of 1,000 people, so there I stuck out even more like a sore thumb … That was painful; nobody ever talked to me unless they had to and I was too shy to initiate conversations with them. So I was completely ignored and that's painful.

(GREEN ET AL., 2005, p. 205)

Guys don't date women who are physically disabled. That's a painful fact. Because this country…, especially young guys, seem to like women who are physically perfect. They like women who are 36-24-36 figures—Barbie dolls…Young guys, they're just not mature enough to look past that.

(GREEN ET AL., 2005, p. 208)

Goffman was working in the interactionist tradition and therefore his work involved the 'micro' study of face-to-face interactions. He was looking at individuals and the problems and dilemmas they faced in living with 'attributes' that were evaluated negatively by others. By doing so, he gave a graphic account of the harm caused to individuals by stigma. He has, however, been taken to task by some critics for the limitations of this 'micro' approach. Inevitably, it put the focus on the labelled and not the labellers. Thus, the focus is on the individual and how they 'manage' stigma. Disabled activists complained that Goffman's work implied that stigma was an 'inevitable' fact of social life offering them few clues as to how to challenge or overcome it (Abberley, 1993). Thus, this type of analysis fails to ask some key questions, such as how stigmatising labels come to be constructed; the values behind them and the discourses that propagate them. This approach can, therefore, divert attention away from the structural causes of stigma.

Several recent authors have argued that Goffman's analysis is incomplete due to this interactionist, 'micro' focus (Link & Phelan, 2001). Tyler and Slater (2018) have suggested that we now need to re-think the concept of stigma in a wider context. Link and Phelan (2001) have suggested that stigma consists of four components:

1) Distinguishing and labelling differences
2) Associating human differences with negative attributes
3) Separating 'us' from 'them'
4) Status loss and discrimination

The first three components mirror the stages described by Becker in labelling theory as well as much of Goffman's work on stigma. It is the final component of their model which draws attention to the discriminatory nature of stigma and its links to social inequalities. Thus, Link and Phelan associate stigma with the existence of inequality and status hierarchies in society. We might expect therefore that more unequal societies will have more in-built systems of discrimination against people who are seen as 'less equal'. Link and Phelan suggest that this **'structural discrimination'** is implicated in the enactment of stigma. Thus, they say that 'all manner of disadvantage can result outside of a model in which one person does something bad to another' (p. 372). There can be institutionalised discrimination against whole classes of people to whom stigmatising labels have been applied. For example, Wacquant (2008) has argued that whole communities, such as those living in social housing, can be neglected and marginalised due to 'territorial stigmatisation' (see Chapter 2). An example from the healthcare field is that stigmatised illnesses, such as schizophrenia, receive less funding for research, treatment or support. We can see the existence of 'Cinderella specialties', such as mental health, rheumatology and elderly care as examples of structural discrimination in healthcare.

Understanding that stigma and labelling may involve institutionalised discrimination that is built in to social structures means that tackling stigma involves a lot more than simply changing the hearts and minds of individuals. Tyler and Slater (2018) have argued that alongside campaigns to alleviate stigma other campaigns exist that deliberately propagate stigmatising ideas and beliefs. Scambler (2018) describes stigma as having been 'weaponised' for social and political ends. Thus, in the era of austerity following the global financial crisis of 2007–2008, a growing political discourse demonised disabled people who were in receipt of incapacity benefits, describing them as 'workshy' and implying that their disabilities could be fake. This had negative effects on attitudes to sick and disabled people generally (Disability Rights UK, 2012). This distracted attention from the real causes of the financial crisis (namely, the reckless actions of financial institutions) while justifying cuts in welfare benefits and encouraging prejudice and moral condemnation of people with disabilities (Tyler & Slater, 2018). Similarly, the policy discourses which highlight the 'problem' of 'bed blockers' and put pressure on health professionals to accelerate patient throughput create the conditions for negative labelling of elderly patients with long-term illnesses (see Chapter 10). We will consider discrimination against disabled people in more detail in the next section.

Living With Disability

THE MEDICAL OR 'PERSONAL TRAGEDY' MODEL

According to the World Health Organization, one billion people worldwide experience some form of disability (WHO, 2011). Defining disability can be a contentious issue. Until recently, disability was medically defined. For example, the WHO (1980) produced the International Classification of Impairments, Disabilities and Handicaps (ICIDH) which medically defined 'impairment', 'disability' and 'handicap'. **Impairment** was defined medically as a physical or psychological loss of structure or function. **Disability** was described as an inability to perform functions considered 'normal' within society due to impairment. **Handicap** was described as the disadvantage that resulted from the impairment and its effect on 'normal' functioning.

The 1960s and 1970s heralded an era in which the civil rights movement sought to reduce inequalities and discrimination in relation to race, gender and other characteristics, such as sexual orientation. For example, Equal Pay Acts requiring women to be paid the same wages as men for the same work were passed in the US in 1963 and in the UK in 1970. Homosexuality was finally legalised in the UK in England and Wales in 1967 and the Race Relations Act banned racial discrimination in 1968. However, due to the medical model of disability, many disabled people still had limited rights to manage their own lives and many were still incarcerated in long-term institutions. Thus, the disabled rights movement developed to challenge institutionalised discrimination against people with disabilities and institutional control over their lives. They demanded that disabled people were given autonomy, equal opportunities and full access to meaningful participation in society. A number of groups were formed by disabled people to fight for their rights often modelled on the US Black civil rights movement. In the UK, these included the Union of the Physically Impaired Against Segregation (UPIAS).

From the 1960s onwards, disability activists started to strongly criticise the biomedical, deficit model of disability employed by organisations, such as the WHO. They described this **medical model** of disability as the **'personal tragedy'** model which portrays people with disabilities as abnormal and pitiable (Oliver, 1990). Similarly, many saw sociological studies of how the disabled 'adjust' to disability as colluding with this personal tragedy model. As we have already seen, people act towards things (or people) according to the meaning they attach to them. The disability rights movement was thus, in many respects, a fight to overthrow the strongly negative labels and stereotypes attached to people with disabilities. Labels are real in their consequences and disability activists believed that the medical model and medical institutions had for too long curbed and controlled the lives of disabled people.

THE SOCIAL MODEL OF DISABILITY

Disability activists proposed a new **'social model'** of disability which recognised the disabled as an oppressed group. According to UPIAS (1976):

> 'Disability is something imposed on top of our impairments by the way we are unnecessarily isolated and excluded from full participation in society. Disabled people are therefore an oppressed group in society.'

The WHO classification system became controversial as disability rights activists started to reject its deficit model of disability demanding instead a model based on the UPIAS definition which acknowledged the social oppression of the disabled. According to UPIAS (1976), disability resulted from the actions of a society that refused to accommodate and include those who were different.

> 'It is necessary to grasp the distinction between the physical impairment and the social situation, called 'disability,' of people with such impairment. Thus, we define impairment as lacking part of or all of a limb, or having a defective limb, organ or mechanism of the body; and disability as the disadvantage or restriction of activity caused by a contemporary social organisation which takes no or little account of people who have physical impairments and thus excludes them from participation in the mainstream of social activities. Physical disability is therefore a particular form of social oppression.'
>
> (UPIAS, 1976)

For example, a person with short stature is only unable to use a lift because the lift engineer has sited the lift button at the height presumed to suit the 'normal' lift user. Similarly, many public and workplace toilets, even in some hospitals, cannot accommodate a wheelchair. Modern industrial society has often been designed in a way that systematically excludes those who differ from what is assumed to be 'normal'.

Thus, disability activists proposed the replacement of the medical model of disability with a **'social model'** of disability (Oliver, 1990, 2013). The social model articulated the disability movement's struggle for equal rights. According to the social model, it was not bodily impairments that prevented the disabled from fully participating in society but the social barriers that had been placed in their way. This focus on social barriers led to campaigns for better access and inclusion which had positive consequences for many disabled people. The model focused attention, firstly, on physical barriers such as access to transport and buildings and secondly, on cultural barriers such as low expectations and patronising and discriminatory attitudes towards people with disabilities. Many people with disabilities faced structural discrimination in all areas of their lives including education, work, housing and leisure.

The social model was important for people with disabilities politically, practically and psychologically (Shakespeare, 2010). It gave people with impairments a new way to understand their situation and offered them a model which could afford them more self-respect and confidence as well as giving them a sense of collective identity. It led to disability rights legislation in the UK and some other countries which placed a responsibility on institutions, such as schools and workplaces, to remove social barriers and facilitate greater access for disabled people. It also kickstarted the independent living movement, which allowed some people with impairments to take control of the services they received through receiving direct payments. This allowed them to manage their own assistance and care (Thomas, 2010). A series of laws have also been passed to protect the rights of people with disabilities, most recently the 2010 Equality Act. This places a responsibility on employers and providers of services, such as education, to make 'reasonable adjustments' to anything that puts a disabled person at a substantial disadvantage compared to someone who is able-bodied. This might include physical barriers to access or policies and procedures that disadvantage people with disabilities. However, efforts to improve the rights of people with disabilities have largely ignored older people who make up a high proportion of people with disabilities, focusing instead on those of working age.

The social model has some limitations. By focusing solely on the role of social barriers in creating disability it downplayed the effects of impairments. Many people with impairments experience pain and suffering as a result of bodily impairments, particularly those with long-term illnesses. The social model worked well for people with a stable, acquired disability, such as loss of a limb, but, perhaps less well, for those with painful progressive illnesses, such as rheumatoid arthritis. Thus, Shakespeare (2017) has rejected the idea that it is only disability (understood as social oppression) that makes impairment a problem to the individual. Bodily impairments, such as pain and fatigue can be burdensome for the individual whether they experience social barriers or not. Feminist disabled writers in particular have argued for the importance of understanding the personal experience of both impairment and disability (Thomas, 2010). Thus, we can conclude that the social model justly criticised the medical model and acted as a powerful political tool that played an important part in tackling social barriers and disability discrimination. However, it does not offer a complete understanding of the experience of disability.

Deprivation and Disability

The disabled rights movement has done a great deal to address disability discrimination. However, very large numbers of people with disabilities still experience poverty, deprivation and poor support. Almost half of the people living in poverty in the UK are disabled or living with someone with a disability. One-third of disabled people live in poverty (JRF, 2022) and large numbers of disabled people are classified as destitute, meaning that they lack the basic necessities of life, such as adequate food and heating (JRF, 2022). In recent years, the benefits provided to disabled people have been steadily eroded as benefit cuts and 'reforms', such as the abolition of Disability Living Allowance, have hit the disabled harder than any other group. This has left a fifth of people with disabilities in 'deep poverty' (see Chapter 2) (JRF, 2022). Ryan (2020) has chronicled the lives of individual people with disabilities hit by cuts in benefits and social care and living in deep poverty and describes situations where people with disabilities have been forced to sell televisions and cookers to pay bills. Levels of malnutrition, as well as levels of debt, have increased amongst people with disabilities. People with disabilities face a higher cost of living and continue to face barriers in access to paid work. The social care services which help people with disabilities to live independently have also been severely cut back (Ryan, 2020).

Negative attitudes towards people with disabilities have also risen in the last decade with an increase of hate crimes directed at people with disabilities (Healy, 2020) The demonisation of people with disabilities on welfare benefits in the press as well as in official policy discourse has fuelled a rise in stigmatisation of the disabled (Garthwaite, 2014). A recent report by disabled groups to the United Nations Committee monitoring UK compliance with the United Nations Convention on the Rights of People with Disabilities, concluded that the situation of disabled people in the UK had worsened during the pandemic. Many disabled people reported that they had felt that they were regarded as 'expendable' and that the pervasive discourse from both government sources and the press was that the deaths of disabled people were less important than the deaths of the able bodied. Some said it now felt 'dangerous' to be disabled (Inclusion London, 2022). Thus, despite some progress in disabled rights, many problems persist.

REFLECTION POINT

Think about your most recent encounter with a patient with a disability in a clinical setting. This could be a physical disability, learning disability or sensory impairment. How well do you think your service provided for the needs of this individual? Was the environment fully accessible for this individual? How could the setting be improved for disabled people?

How well did staff communicate with the individual? What did you notice about staff attitudes and behaviours? Did you notice any differences in how the individual was treated when compared to an able-bodied patient? What do you think the reasons for these differences were?

Summary of Key Points

- Interactionist studies exploring the experience of long-term illness have shown a number of ways in which long-term conditions disrupt people's everyday life.
- There is increasing pressure on patients to self-manage their condition. There is, as yet, limited evidence regarding the efficacy of self-management, and it may place excessive demands on some patients.
- People with long-term illnesses and disability may suffer stigma, status loss, social exclusion and discrimination.
- Disability rights activists have criticised the medical model of disability for restricting the lives of disabled people.
- The 'social model' of disability focuses on addressing social barriers to allow the disabled full participation in society.

Further Reading

Goffman, E. (2009). *Stigma: Notes on the management of spoiled identity*. Simon and Schuster.

Inclusion London. (2022). *United Nations convention on the rights of disabled people: Westminster Government Civil Society Shadow report*. Retrieved January 17, 2024, from https://www.inclusionlondon.org.uk/wp-content/uploads/2022/03/Westminster-Government-Civil-Society-Shadow-Report.pdf.

Link, B. G., & Phelan, J. C. (2001). Conceptualizing stigma. *Annual Review of Sociology, 27*, 363–385.

Oliver, M. (2013). The social model of disability: Thirty years on. *Disability & Society, 28*(7), 1024–1026.

References

Abberley, P. (1993). Disabled people and normality. In Hurst, R., Swain, J., Finkelstein, V., French, S., & Oliver, M. (Eds.), *Disabling barriers—Enabling environments* (pp. 107–115). Sage Publications.

Apesoa-Varano, E. C., Barker, J. C., & Hinton, L. (2015). Shards of sorrow: Older men's accounts of their depression experience. *Social Science & Medicine, 124*, 1–8.

Becker, H. (2008). *Outsiders*. Simon and Schuster.

Becker, H. (2018). Labelling theory reconsidered. In McIntosh, M., & Rock, P. (Eds.), *Deviance and Social Control* (pp. 41–66). Routledge.

Bennett, B. L., Buchanan, W. W., & Harden, R. M. (1972). Rheumatology-the 'Cinderella' specialty: An examination of doctors' attitudes to training and careers. *Medical Education, 6*(3), 232–237.

Bibby, J., Everest, G., & Abbs, I. (2020). *Will COVID-19 be a watershed moment for health inequalities*. The Health Foundation.

Blumer, H. (1986). *Symbolic interactionism: Perspective and method*. University of California Press.

Borrell, C., Palència, L., Muntaner, C., Urquía, M., Malmusi, D., & O'Campo, P. (2014). Influence of macro-social policies on women's health and gender inequalities in health. *Epidemiologic Reviews, 36*(1), 31–48.

Bury, M. (1982). Chronic illness as biographical disruption. *Sociology of Health & illness, 4*(2), 167–182.

Cayton, H. (2006). The flat-pack patient? Creating health together. *Patient Education and Counseling, 62*(3), 288–290.

Charmaz, K. (1983). Loss of self: A fundamental form of suffering in the chronically ill. *Sociology of Health & Illness, 5*(2), 168–195.

Charmaz, K. (2020). Experiencing stigma and exclusion: The influence of neoliberal perspectives, practices, and policies on living with chronic illness and disability. *Symbolic Interaction, 43*(1), 21–45.

Collins, K. (2005). Cold, cold housing and respiratory illnesses. In Nicol, F., & Rudge, J. (Eds.), *Cutting the cost of cold: Affordable warmth for healthier homes* (pp. 49–60). Routledge.

Corbin, J., & Strauss, A. (1985). Managing chronic illness at home: Three lines of work. *Qualitative Sociology, 8*(3), 224–247.

Corbin, J. M. (1998). The Corbin and Strauss chronic illness trajectory model: An update. *Research and Theory for Nursing Practice, 12*(1), 33.

Corbin, JM., & Strauss, A. (1991). A nursing model for chronic illness management based upon the trajectory framework. *Scholarly Inquiry for Nursing Practice, 5*(3), 155–174.

Cowie, L., Morgan, M., White, P., & Gulliford, M. (2009). Experience of continuity of care of patients with multiple long-term conditions in England. *Journal of Health Services Research & Policy, 14*(2), 82–87.

Cresswell, M. (2020). Self-harm and moral codes in emergency departments in England. *Social Theory & Health, 18*(3), 257–269.

Davis, J. M., & Watson, N. (2001). Where are the children's experiences? Analysing social and cultural exclusion in 'special' and 'mainstream' schools. *Disability & Society, 16*(5), 671–687.

Department of Health. (2004). *The NHS improvement plan: Putting people at the heart of public services*. The Stationery Office.

Disability Rights UK. (2012). *Press portrayal of disabled people. A rise in hostility fuelled by austerity?* Disability Rights UK.

Donaldson, L. (2003). Expert patients usher in a new era of opportunity for the NHS: The expert patient programme will improve the length and quality of lives. *BMJ, 326*(7402), 1279–1280.

Dorling, D. (2011). *So you think you know about Britain?* Hachette.

Garthwaite, K. (2014). Fear of the brown envelope: Exploring welfare reform with long-term sickness benefits recipients. *Social Policy & Administration, 48*(7), 782–798.

Goffman, E. (2009). *Stigma: Notes on the management of spoiled identity*. Simon and Schuster.

Green, S., Davis, C., Karshmer, E., Marsh, P., & Straight, B. (2005). Living stigma: The impact of labelling, stereotyping, separation, status loss, and discrimination in the lives of individuals with disabilities and their families. *Sociological Inquiry, 75*(2), 197–215.

Greenhalgh, T. (2009). Patient and public involvement in chronic illness: Beyond the expert patient. *BMJ, 338*, 629–631.

Griffin, S. (2022). Emergency care is in "dire" situation after loss of NHS beds, says Royal College. *BMJ, 377*, o1376.

Griffiths, L. (2001). Categorising to exclude: The discursive construction of cases in community mental health teams. *Sociology of Health & Illness, 23*(5), 678–700.

Hatch, S. L., Frissa, S., Verdecchia, M., Stewart, R., Fear, N. T., Reichenberg, A., Morgan, C., Kankulu, B., Clark, J., Gazard, B., & Medcalf, R. (2011). Identifying socio-demographic and socioeconomic determinants of health inequalities in a diverse London community: The South East London Community Health (SELCoH) study. *BMC Public Health, 11*, 1–17.

Hayanga, B., Stafford, M., Saunders, C. L., & Bécares, L. (2022). *Ethnic inequalities in age-related patterns of multiple long-term conditions in England: Analysis of primary care and nationally representative survey data*. medRxiv.

Healy, J. C. (2020). It spreads like a creeping disease': Experiences of victims of disability hate crimes in austerity Britain. *Disability & Society, 35*(2), 176–200.

Hinder, S., & Greenhalgh, T. (2012). "This does my head in". Ethnographic study of self-management by people with diabetes. *BMC Health Services Research, 12*, 83.

Inclusion London. (2022). *United Nations convention on the rights of disabled people: Westminster Government Civil Society Shadow report.* Retrieved January 17, 2024, from https://www.inclusionlondon.org.uk/wp-content/uploads/2022/03/Westminster-Government-Civil-Society-Shadow-Report.pdf.

Jeffery, R. (1979). Normal rubbish: Deviant patients in casualty departments. *Sociology of Health & illness, 1*(1), 90–107.

Johnson, M., & Webb, C. (1995). Rediscovering unpopular patients: The concept of social judgement. *Journal of Advanced Nursing, 21*(3), 466–475.

Jowsey, T., & Yen, L. (2012). Time spent on health related activities associated with chronic illness: A scoping literature review. *BMC Public Health, 12*(1), 1–12.

Jowsey, T., Dennis, S., Yen, L., Mofizul Islam, M., Parkinson, A., & Dawda, P. (2016). Time to manage: Patient strategies for coping with an absence of care coordination and continuity. *Sociology of Health & Illness, 38*(6), 854–873.

JRF. (2022). *UK poverty 2022: The essential guide to understanding poverty in the UK.* Retrieved January 17, 2024, from https://www.jrf.org.uk/report/uk-poverty-2022.

Kings Fund. (2013). *Long term conditions and multi morbidity.* Retrieved January 17, 2024, from https://www.kingsfund.org.uk/projects/time-think-differently/trends-disease-and-disability-long-term-conditions-multi-morbidity.

Latimer, J. (1997). Giving patients a future: The constituting of classes in an acute medical unit. *Sociology of Health & Illness, 19*(2), 160–185.

Link, B. G., & Phelan, J. C. (2001). Conceptualizing stigma. *Annual Review of Sociology, 27*, 363–385.

Lorig, K. R., & Holman, H. R. (2003). Self-management education: History, definition, outcomes, and mechanisms. *Annals of Behavioral Medicine, 26*(1), 1–7.

Malmusi, D., Artazcoz, L., Benach, J., & Borrell, C. (2012). Perception or real illness? How chronic conditions contribute to gender inequalities in self-rated health. *The European Journal of Public Health, 22*(6), 781–786.

McDonald, R., Rogers, A., & Macdonald, W. (2008). Dependence and identity: Nurses and chronic conditions in a primary care setting. *Journal of Health Organization and Management, 22*(3), 294–308.

Miller, W. R., Von Gaudecker, J., Tanner, A., & Buelow, J. M. (2020). Epilepsy self-management during a pandemic: Experiences of people with epilepsy. *Epilepsy & Behavior, 111*, 107238.

Nemiroff, L. (2022). We can do better: Addressing ageism against older adults in healthcare. *Healthcare Management Forum, 35*(2), 118–122.

Newbould, J., Taylor, D., & Bury, M. (2006). Lay-led self-management in chronic illness: A review of the evidence. *Chronic Illness, 2*(4), 249–261.

Oliver, M. (1990). *The Politics of Disablement.* Macmillan.

Oliver, M. (2013). The social model of disability: Thirty years on. *Disability & Society, 28*(7), 1024–1026.

Perry, A., Lawrence, V., & Henderson, C. (2020). Stigmatisation of those with mental health conditions in the acute general hospital setting: A qualitative framework synthesis. *Social Science & Medicine, 255*, 112974.

Potter, C. M., Kelly, L., Hunter, C., Fitzpatrick, R., & Peters, M. (2018). The context of coping: A qualitative exploration of underlying inequalities that influence health services support for people living with long-term conditions. *Sociology of Health & Illness, 40*(1), 130–145.

Ryan, F. (2020). *Crippled: Austerity and the demonization of disabled people.* Verso Books.

Saunders, B. (2017). 'It seems like you're going around in circles': Recurrent biographical disruption constructed through the past, present and anticipated future in the narratives of young adults with inflammatory bowel disease. *Sociology of Health & Illness, 39*(5), 726–740.

Scambler, G. (2018). Heaping blame on shame: 'Weaponising stigma' for neoliberal times. *The Sociological Review, 66*(4), 766–782.

Scott, R. A. (2017). *The making of blind men: A study of adult socialization.* Routledge.

Shakespeare, T. (2010). The social model of disability. In L. J. Davis (Ed.), *The Disability Studies Reader* (pp. 266–273). Routledge.

Shakespeare, T. (2017). Critiquing the social model. In E. Emens (Ed.), *Disability and Equality Law* (pp. 67–94). Routledge.

Stockwell F. (1972). *The unpopular patient.* Royal College of Nursing.

Strudwick, R. M (2016). Labelling patients. *Radiography, 22*(1), 50–55.

Tausig, M. (2013). The sociology of chronic illness and self-care management. In J. J. Kronenfeld (Ed.), *Social determinants, health disparities and linkages to health and health care* (pp. 247–272). Emerald Group Publishing.

Thomas, C. (2010). Medical sociology and disability theory. In Scambler, G (Ed.), *New directions in the sociology of chronic and disabling conditions: Assaults on the lifeworld* (pp. 37–56). Palgrave Macmillan.

Tower, M., Rowe, J., & Wallis, M. (2012). Investigating patients' experiences: Methodological usefulness of interpretive interactionism. *Nurse Researcher, 20*(1), 39–44.

Tyler, I., & Slater, T. (2018). Rethinking the sociology of stigma. *The Sociological Review, 66*(4), 721–743.

UPIAS. (1976). *Fundamental Principles of disability*. Retrieved January 16, 2024, from https://the-ndaca.org/resources/audio-described-gallery/fundamental-principles-of-disability/.

Valdez, A. (2021). Words matter: Labelling, bias and stigma in nursing. *Journal of Advanced Nursing, 77*(11), e33–e35.

Wacquant, L. (2008). Territorial stigmatization in the age of advanced marginality. In Houtsonen, J., & Antikainen, A. (Eds.), *Symbolic power in cultural contexts: Uncovering social reality* (pp. 43–52). Brill.

Williams, G. (1984). The genesis of chronic illness: Narrative re construction. *Sociology of Health & Illness, 6*(2), 175–200.

Williams, S. (2001). Chronic illness as biographical disruption or biographical disruption as chronic illness? Reflections on a core concept. *Sociology of Health & Illness, 22*(1), 40–67.

Williams, G. (2002). Chronic illness and the pursuit of virtue in everyday life. In Radley, A. (Ed.), *Worlds of illness: Biographical and Cultural Perspectives on Health and Disease Routledge* (pp. 104–120).

Wohland, P., Rees, P., Nazroo, J., & Jagger, C. (2015). Inequalities in healthy life expectancy between ethnic groups in England and Wales in 2001. *Ethnicity & Health, 20*(4), 341–353.

World Health Organization. (1980). *International classification of impairments, disabilities, and handicaps: A manual of classification relating to the consequences of disease, published in accordance with resolution WHA29. 35 of the Twenty-ninth World Health Assembly*. World Health Organization.

World Health Organization. (2011). *World report on disability 2011*. Retrieved January 17, 2024, from https://www.who.int/teams/noncommunicable-diseases/sensory-functions-disability-and-rehabilitation/world-report-on-disability.

PART 3

The Social and Political Organisation of Healthcare

Healthcare Policy and Organisational Change

Introduction

This chapter will look firstly at healthcare policies and how they are made. It will consider how sociological and political theories can help us to understand how and why healthcare policy gets made. It will examine what health policy is and who makes it. It will also outline the key political ideologies that have underpinned health policies in the UK and the global context within which policy is made.

The chapter will then look in detail at the development of the National Health Service (NHS). It will briefly describe what healthcare was like before the NHS; how the National Health Service developed; the cascade of organisational changes that occurred in the NHS between the 1980s and 2010s and the structure of the NHS following the 2022 Health and Social Care Act. It will review the impact of these organisational changes on key policy issues and challenges. This chapter is complemented by the final two chapters of the book which cover changes in healthcare professional work and changing places of care.

WHAT IS HEALTH POLICY?

When we talk about policies we refer to plans or ideas that have either been collectively agreed upon by an institution/group or mandated by people in power. Policies can work horizontally to coordinate the actions of a group of people or they can work vertically as a set of rules imposed on a group of people by those with power; the latter is more commonplace (Colebatch, 2009). Policies set out what to do in particular situations.

Policies can be small scale and local or they can encompass a national institution, such as the NHS. An example of a local policy is a policy for reporting an 'adverse incident', such as a fall. This policy should tell staff exactly what they should and should not report; what data they need to record; who they should report the incident to and what will happen to the data. It should also cover what both the local organisation and wider NHS will do to learn from the incident and prevent future harm (Mahajan, 2010). For a policy to be successful it needs to be **clear** and **understandable**. It also needs to be **achievable** and this means that people need access to the means (time, resources and training) to deliver it. Policies need to have **clear aims** which users can understand and indicate **how success will be measured**; for example, a reduction in patient safety incidents. Policymakers often fail to adequately address these policy essentials. Thus, studies have shown that lack of clarity in incident reporting policies and a lack of feedback on the outcomes of reporting have acted as barriers to reporting adverse incidents. This suggests that existing policies have not been fully successful (Bovis et al., 2018).

Other authors have suggested that a policy should not contradict or conflict with other policies. It is also important that staff and organisations are not overloaded with too many policies or frequent policy changes. As we will see shortly, when we look at the organisation of the NHS, politicians have often ignored this advice. The NHS has often been overloaded with frequent organisational changes and multiple, short-lived, conflicting policies (Paton, 2016). Policymakers have often failed to clearly explain how a policy will work; with some policies little more than a vague 'bright idea'. This leaves health service staff having to try to flesh out the details of implementation on the ground. This process has been called **'manipulated emergence'** (Harrison & Wood, 1999).

When we talk about health policy in the NHS, we are usually talking about much wider scale changes involving changes in laws or in the directions given by governments to healthcare institutions. In recent years, these have often involved wholesale reorganisation of services; sometimes described by critics as **'re-disorganisation'** (Paton, 2023). Looi and Kisely (2019) suggest that these frequent policy changes are designed to prove politicians and senior managers are 'doing something' and to give an illusion of progress, but that they are dysfunctional for both clinical staff and patients. Before going on to look at these recent policy changes in the NHS, we will consider what social and political theorists have said about how health policy gets made at the national level and who makes it.

How Policy Gets Made and Who Makes It

Firstly, policymaking was traditionally believed to follow a **'rational' model**. This was seen as a logical process in which 'policymakers' identified a problem; reviewed alternative responses to the problem; consulted interested parties; evaluated the evidence about what worked best; implemented a change and then evaluated what had worked. While policymaking is still often presented as a rational process, sadly, the reality of policymaking is often very far from this rational model for various, usually political, reasons (Colebatch, 2009).

A **second** model of policymaking suggests that it is governed by **'bounded rationality'**. This means that policymaking operates with a limited range of vision and some evidence is simply not admitted to the policy process. Politics in its widest sense influences what are recognised as problems and what solutions to problems are allowed onto the political agenda. Governments often claim to be delivering evidence-based policy and doing 'what works'. However, governments are usually highly selective in their choice of evidence and actively try to shape the evidence available. For example, during the COVID-19 pandemic, governments claimed to be 'following the science' in their policy decisions. However, what this meant in practice was that they sought the advice of scientists whose views they found politically palatable, while ignoring other evidence and scientific opinion. Arguably, this narrowness of vision led to a large number of policy mistakes; for example, the decision at the very start of the pandemic that closing the UK border to travellers from China was not necessary caused a large amount of preventable transmission of the virus into the UK (Cairney, 2021). The proceedings of the COVID-19 inquiry have also suggested that even the advice that politicians were given by insiders was also often ignored and that decision-making was frequently chaotic (Sridhar, 2023).

Politics and politicians can also shape the availability of evidence leading to **policy-based evidence**. Most policy research is funded by governments or political parties who want to shape the policy agenda or groups with a particular vested interest, such as the tobacco lobby. These people have been called 'policy entrepreneurs' (Cairney, 2019). Thus, following the evidence or 'science' is constrained by the tendency to fund the production of politically sponsored research leading to a shortage of robust, independent evidence. This is compounded by a tendency to ignore outsider voices. This insider bias by a narrow policy elite results in the exclusion of dissenting voices and policy options are confined within narrow (often ideological) tramlines (Paton, 2016). This process also tends to exclude minority groups and thus it reinforces inequalities. We looked in Chapter 2 at the sociologist Max Weber's theory that inequality consisted of disparities of class (economic position), status and power. In the policymaking arena, we can see these inequalities of power at work, rendering some groups voiceless. While some groups are simply not heard, selective powerful groups and organisations are favoured and have their voices amplified.

The **third** and most influential policymaking model is the **'policy streams'** approach (Kingdon, 1993). Kingdon said that there are **three 'streams' of activity** that lead to policy being made. When these three streams come together they create a **window of opportunity** in which policy change can happen. Windows of opportunity often happen as the result of high-profile media attention to a particular issue. As media attention is often short lived, many problems and their solutions will miss their window of opportunity and policy change will not happen.

The first stream is the **'policy problem stream'**, and it is here that situations get defined as problems and do or do not make it onto the policymaking agenda. Kingdon suggests that debates about a problem take place among **'problem entrepreneurs'** who try to draw attention to a problem and champion their definition of it. Problem entrepreneurs may include professionals, charities, patient groups, commercial firms, academics, celebrities, media organisations and politicians. How a problem is defined and the status of the people championing it influences whether a policy gets onto the political agenda or not. Without influential backers and politically acceptable arguments it is difficult to get a problem on the policy agenda even when there is compelling evidence for change.

Examples: Getting an Issue Onto the Policy Agenda

Groups representing the 1.5 million women with endometriosis have highlighted the problem of late diagnosis and poor access to treatment and used the media to try to draw attention to this problem. There has been sporadic media interest in this issue and some government acknowledgment of the problem in the Women's Health Strategy (Department of Health and Social Care, 2022). However, there has been no concrete policy change (Seear, 2016).

By contrast, treatment of the menopause has been the topic of a high-profile media campaign, with the support of celebrities, such as Davina McCall. This campaign led to concrete policy changes to improve the availability of hormone replacement therapy and reduce its cost. Orgad and Rottenberg (2023) have suggested that this 'menopause moment' came about because of its high-profile sponsors and also because it was framed in an individualistic discourse of self-improvement which incorporated economic arguments about improving women's workplace productivity. The campaign also encouraged the consumption of 'wellness' products and thus drew the support of commercial interests including the pharmaceutical industry. They suggest that policy change occurred, firstly, because the problem and its solution were framed within a politically acceptable discourse and, secondly, because the campaign was able to mobilise some powerful interest groups.

The **second** stream is the **'policy solution stream'**. Here, those people that Kingdon calls **'policy entrepreneurs'** promote their own pet solutions to problems. Policy entrepreneurs may be academics, politicians or commercial organisations, who have something to gain from promoting a particular solution, for example, firms of management consultants. There may also be some overlap between problem entrepreneurs and policy entrepreneurs. There are a number of organisations that act as policy entrepreneurs including 'think tanks', such as the King's Fund, the Nuffield Foundation and political campaigning groups. Policy entrepreneurs often promote the same solution to a wide range of problems and this often has a strongly ideological focus; for example, the promotion of neoliberal ideas, such as outsourcing to the private sector to solve NHS problems, such as staff shortages (Hoefer, 2022). These groups may also promote fashionable management ideas (or 'fads'), such as 'leadership' or 'lean' management (Hewison & Griffiths, 2004).

The final stream is the **political stream**. It is in the political arena that the political will to address a problem either gains momentum or dissipates. Kingdon says that this political stream will only exist for a short time before the problem fades from the political and media agenda. This is the **policy window**. The policy window will often close without any action being taken. A policy window can open as a result of sustained research and campaigning or because a high-profile case in the media has led to a **'moral panic'** about an issue. Moral panics lead to demands for greater regulation of particular situations, behaviours, things or people. The sociological theory of **'moral panic'** refers to heightened public concern about an issue that is volatile and disproportionate (Goode & Ben-Yehuda, 2010). Importantly, a moral panic normally also involves negative moral judgements about particular groups or behaviours; for example, the moral panic about obesity has increased support for punitive anti-obesity policies which 'bludgeon the vulnerable' (Mannion & Small, 2019, p. 683). Policy made on the back of a moral panic is often hasty and badly thought out.

The **political stream** is the most unpredictable and often the least rational part of the policy process. Whether policy gets enacted often depends on the media's framing of a problem as well as politicians' ideological beliefs, and their calculations about the effect of a policy on their own political fortunes. Calnan (2020) says that the media's framing of a problem is often biased and frequently represents vested interests. We can see, therefore, that in many circumstances, evidence only plays a minor role in the production of policy. Health professionals who want to get an issue onto the policy agenda need to do more than provide evidence that change is needed; they also need to be politically astute to get politicians to listen (Traynor, 2013). There can be extremely good evidence in favour of a policy yet it may never make it onto the political agenda. Yet, policy is too often made on the basis of weak or non-existent evidence.

REFLECTION POINT

Think of a policy change that you think could solve a problem with patient care. How do you think health professionals could get this problem onto the political agenda?

POLITICAL PHILOSOPHIES INFORMING HEALTH POLICIES

We have said that political philosophies (ideologies) have an important influence on health policy and will now briefly outline the two key political ideologies that have informed UK health policy. It is the tension between these two political ideologies that has created much of the turbulence in UK health policy and organisational structures since the 1980s.

Social Democracy

Social democracy was influenced by twentieth century ethical socialist thinkers, such as Tawney (1952), who sought to achieve social justice through gradual democratic reform. The term *social democracy* is used to describe a form of managed capitalism in which the state acts to protect the welfare of the whole population from the risks and insecurities that an unregulated capitalist economy creates for ordinary people. Typically, this includes some state management of the economy to promote economic stability and create high levels of employment. It also includes regulation of private industry in the interests of the whole population; for example, through protecting employees' rights and through environmental and public health legislation. The state also acts to protect the health and welfare of the population through compulsory social insurance which funds insurance-based benefits, such as the state pension and maternity pay, as well as providing a safety net of non-contributory welfare payments for the sick, disabled, unemployed etc. Finally, the state provides publicly funded social services, such as education and healthcare. Social democracy also tries to achieve a modest reduction in inequalities by 'progressive' taxation which takes proportionately higher taxes from those with the most wealth.

The overall aim of social democracy is to mitigate the destructive effects of unregulated capitalism and to promote a sense of community, social cohesion and social stability (Garland, 2016). It was these social democratic ideas that informed the creation of the welfare state after World War II and underpinned the creation of the NHS. Social democracy is informed by ideas of human rights, freedom and social justice but crucially this also includes 'social rights', such as the right to adequate food, housing, education and health (UN General Assembly, 1948). Social democracy declined in popularity among many politicians and economists in the 1970s when it was perceived as unable to handle the economic shocks created by the oil crisis that followed the Arab–Israeli war of 1973. Many welfare institutions built on social democratic principles, such as the NHS, have continued to exist, but since the 1980s, many have found themselves subject to continuing political attack (Garland, 2016).

Neoliberalism

Neoliberalism is a project to reinstate the economic ideas of eighteenth century 'liberal' economists, such as Adam Smith. In economics, the term 'liberal' is used to mean granting more freedom to private finance and enabling the 'free market'. It does not necessarily mean liberalism in terms of political and social freedoms. Neoliberal economic policies have often been accompanied by an increase in authoritarianism, indicated, for example, by large increases in prison populations and greater restrictions on the right to protest. The most influential neoliberal thinker was Hayek (2009) who condemned the welfare state as the 'road to serfdom'. Neoliberalism has been the dominant ideology in UK politics since the Thatcher government of the 1980s. Neoliberalism seeks to undo social democratic reforms and uses the state to restore market 'freedoms'. Thus, Margaret Thatcher committed her government to 'rolling back' the welfare state; reducing controls on private industry; cutting taxation and making taxation less 'progressive' (Steger & Roy, 2010).

According to Steger and Roy (2010) neoliberalism is not just an **ideology**; it is also a **mode of governance** and a **policy package**. The fundamental **ideology** of neoliberalism is individualism. Neoliberals believe that human nature is essentially selfish and that society is made up of competitive individuals pursuing their own economic interests. For neoliberals this is a good thing as they believe in what Adam Smith called the 'invisible hand' (Smith, 2008) of the market; a metaphor for the positive effects that neoliberals believe can accrue from encouraging unfettered self-interest and the introduction of competitive markets into all areas of life (Steger & Roy, 2010). Thus, a key concept justifying neoliberal policies is 'trickle-down economics'. This is the belief that applying pro-market policies that disproportionately favour the wealthy will produce economic benefits that 'trickle down' to everyone else. Research by Hope and Limberg (2020) has suggested that there is little or no credible evidence for this theory.

When we talk about a **mode of governance** we are referring to the ways of thinking, character traits and power relations that neoliberalism promotes. As a mode of governance, it promotes reforms that encourage individualism, competitiveness and commercial self-interest. This also leads to the creation of low-trust institutions that assume that everyone is 'out for themselves'. Neoliberalism distrusts ideas, such as public service, vocation and the public good; seeing them either as fictions or as the enemies of economic growth.

As a **policy package**, neoliberalism promotes several key policy ideas; deregulation of the private sector; privatisation (or failing that commercialisation) of state services; a reduction in welfare benefits and social services; a reduction in employment rights; the removal of controls on the flow of money and finally tax cuts that disproportionately favour the wealthy (Steger & Roy, 2010).

In public services, neoliberalism has been delivered by implementing the tenets of 'new public management' which are described in detail in Chapter 9. In the NHS, this has resulted in successive waves of reform and reorganisation to introduce managerialism, 'modernisation' and 'marketisation'. Critics of neoliberal ideas hold it responsible for the 2008 financial crash; the decline in public services; deepening inequalities and an acceleration of the climate crisis (Sayer, 2014).

THE GLOBAL CONTEXT OF HEALTH POLICIES

Health policies that are decided at a national level have to be understood in a wider global context. In the first place, national governments have to respond to public health issues with a global reach, such as climate change, population displacement and the global spread of infectious diseases, such as COVID-19. Supranational health bodies, such as the World Health Organisation, have sought to influence global health policy through research, aid and advice. However, it is the increased involvement in health policy matters of international economic bodies, such as the World Bank, World Trade Organisation and International Monetary Fund that has increasingly constrained the independence of national governments when setting their countries' health policies (Lister, 2005).

It has thus been suggested that a global elite, largely based in the US, has sought to shape national health agendas through these economic bodies. These bodies have predominantly promoted neoliberal policies, such as managerialism, managed care and the promotion of health markets (Lister, 2005). Multinational corporations can also exercise considerable influence over health policies. For example, they may attempt to subvert public health policies that affect their products, such as policies designed to reduce alcohol consumption (Hastings, 2012). In addition, global management consultancies and global accountancy firms have played a growing role in national healthcare systems. In particular, the US management consultancy McKinsey and Co. has held a substantial number of multimillion-pound contracts with the NHS and some authors have argued that it has exercised undue influence over NHS policy (Davies, 2012).

One of the key exports from the US, promoted by multinational corporations, has been the concept of 'managed care'. In the US, most people have private health insurance through their workplace and their insurance companies pay for-profit providers. However, few people have comprehensive coverage; many are either uninsured or underinsured. The government Medicare and Medicaid programmes provide access to care for the old and those too poor to afford insurance. Neither system provides universal coverage. Managed care was introduced in the US in the 1970s to address specific problems with care costs in the US system. US healthcare costs are far higher than costs in other high-income countries, while public health outcomes remain poor. The traditional US 'fee for service' model was believed to give private hospitals a perverse incentive to carry out more procedures. Thus, insurers introduced 'Health Maintenance Organisations' (HMOs) which gave a flat-rate payment per patient and incentives to providers to reduce care costs.

There was a backlash against managed care in the US in the 1990s due to concerns that it had increased inequalities, restricted choice and diminished access to care (Maynard & Bloor, 1998). This led to the creation of a new version of managed care called 'Accountable Care Organisations' (ACOs) as a result of Obama's Affordable Care Act. ACOs are groups of hospital, primary care and community providers who are given incentives to improve care quality and to control costs. These provider groups are allowed to keep a share of any cost 'savings' that they produce (Pollock & Roderick, 2018). The ACO model has been promoted around the world by US-based multi-national organisations although serious doubts remain as to its relevance to universal, publicly funded, non-profit healthcare systems. However, the UK Health and Care Act, 2022 has introduced the ACO model into the NHS (Pollock & Roderick, 2018).

In the next section we will look at the development of the NHS from its inception to its current structure and, when doing so, need to bear in mind the increasing influence of these global organisations in shaping recent NHS policies.

The Origins of the NHS

HEALTHCARE BEFORE THE NHS

The NHS was created after World War II and built on the Emergency Medical Service that had been put in place to manage casualties during the war. Prior to the war, there had been a patchwork of public, private and charitable health services, but there had been many gaps in provision particularly for the less well off. Workhouses (see Chapter 10) had been formally discontinued in 1930 but continued to exist until 1948 and conditions in these, and their infirmaries for the sick poor, were often grim. A few local councils ran hospitals and these existed alongside charitable 'voluntary hospitals'. Some limited social insurance had been introduced in 1911 which gave working people access to GP services, but this did not cover non-working people or children. For many families, the illness of a child was a financial disaster. In his autobiography, 91-year-old Harry Leslie Smith (2014) described his parent's struggle to care for his young sister who was dying of tuberculosis at home. The family was eventually unable to afford to keep her at home, so his parents pawned their best clothes to pay for her to go into the local workhouse infirmary where she died alone.

Average male life expectancy at this time was 58, and 1 in 20 infants died before their first birthday, so throughout the 1930s there was increasing concern about the poor health of the UK population (Webster, 2002). An investigation into the state of the UK's health services just before the outbreak of war found that there was a chaotic 'patchwork' of services with many gaps in service provision. It also found that there were too many 'profit-making concerns' selling ineffective remedies that took advantage of the 'ignorance and credulity' of the public (Herbert, 1939). It was clear that UK health services were not fit for the future and required major reform.

THE CREATION OF THE POST-WAR WELFARE STATE

In 1942, the Liberal politician, William Beveridge, produced a report which contained a blueprint for social policy after the end of the war following social democratic principles. He envisaged a coherent plan to tackle what he called the **'five giant evils'** of **'idleness, ignorance, disease, squalor and want'**. Tackling these five evils would involve a coordinated approach to reducing unemployment; improving and expanding state education; creating a national health service; building more social housing; regulating private landlords and, finally, providing welfare benefits to reduce poverty, particularly among children. Published in the darkest days of the war (the German 'Blitzkrieg' bombing of British civilians was at its height in 1942), the report promised a better world after the fighting was over. The report was hugely popular with the public although Churchill and his government worried about a negative reception from the US government (National Archives, 2017). After the war, the 1946 Labour government implemented much of the Beveridge Report. This report provided the foundation for the post-war welfare state including the creation of the NHS (Timmins, 2017).

THE CREATION OF THE NHS

In 1944, the wartime coalition government published a white paper promising to create a national health service after the war. There were still arguments within the government as to what form this would take. Should it just provide services for poor people who could not afford medical care or should it be a universal service? The Labour Party had strongly argued for universality and, in 1945, it won a landslide election victory. It set out plans for a universal service in the 1946 National Health Service Act under the direction of Aneurin Bevan, the new Minister of Health (Kynaston, 2008).

The NHS was founded in July 1948. Its aim was to ensure that everyone, regardless of age, gender or economic means (ethnicity was not mentioned) should have access to the best possible healthcare. The aim was to provide a comprehensive service (including both mental and physical health) covering medical and 'allied' services, such as nursing, dentistry and physiotherapy with free access to the necessary medication. The service would promote a 'new attitude' to health by promoting good health rather than just treating illness. The service was to be available to everyone 'irrespective of means' and to be free at the point of use (Ministry of Health, 1944). Britain was the first country in the world to offer free healthcare to the entire population (Timmins, 2017).

Key Features of the 1948 NHS

- It was a universal, comprehensive service.
- The service was free to everyone at the point of use and was funded through taxation and, to a smaller extent, national insurance contributions.
- It was a truly national service; individuals had a right to treatment anywhere in the UK.
- The service was coordinated through 14 regional hospital boards overseen by the Ministry of Health.
- Hospital services, primary care and community services were organised through three separate 'arms' of the service. Hospitals were run by Hospital Boards, community services, such as district nursing, were run by local councils and primary care services were run by Executive Councils.

The NHS was created during a time of post-war austerity, so initial spending was low, and the service overspent in its first 2 years. There were a number of reasons for this; in the first place, the start of the NHS uncovered a great deal of unmet need, particularly for dentures for the toothless and spectacles for people who had been 'fumbling around' all their lives in spectacles bought from Woolworth's (Kynaston, 2008). Secondly, the start of the NHS uncovered the poor state of many UK hospitals; many were bomb damaged and most over 100 years old. After this, spending on the NHS declined through the 1950s and lagged well behind other Western nations. The Guillebaud inquiry into NHS spending in 1956 concluded that the NHS was extremely efficient but was underfunded (Ministry of Health, 1956).

In spite of this frugality, the initial overspending in the first 2 years had created an enduring narrative among opponents of a universal system that the NHS was a 'bottomless pit' of spending (Webster, 2002). The other argument against a universal NHS, that has been around since its beginning, is that the NHS is used (or 'abused') by the 'wrong' sort of people. This is a discourse that **'others'** the disadvantaged, particularly the poor and ethnic minorities. The Liverpool Echo complained of 'coloured people' using the service and an article in the Manchester Guardian, drawing on eugenic ideas, complained that the NHS would end 'selective elimination' and lead to an increase in 'congenitally deformed' and 'feckless' people. This implied that the babies of the poor should continue to be allowed to die in childhood to eliminate the 'feckless' (Kynaston, 2008). This narrative about the undeserving welfare 'scrounger' abusing services would become increasingly prevalent in the twenty-first century, but was being articulated at the dawn of the NHS by those who opposed its principle of universality.

The NHS remained stable throughout the 1950s and 1960s. Spending remained low, but there was some modest investment, and services were improved and modernised. The principle of a universal service free at the point of need had gained enduring support with the public and the NHS became a cherished institution (Cohen, 2020). In 1974, the first major reorganisation of the service took place, instigated by the Conservative government of Edward Heath who hired the US management consultancy, McKinsey and Co., to redesign the service (Levitt, 1976). It added 'team management' to the service with several new tiers of management. Disillusionment with the new, top-heavy structure was rapid. It marked the early beginnings of an era that has been described as 'continuous revolution' (Webster, 2002) in which successive governments and 'policy entrepreneurs' have used the NHS as an experimental laboratory for testing out different neoliberal ideas about how to run public services.

REFLECTION POINT

Look back over the original aims of the NHS described in the section above. Do you agree with these aims? Do you think these aims should still apply to the NHS today?

Reform and Reorganisation: The Era of Continuous Revolution

THATCHER AND THE 'GRIFFITHS' REFORMS

When Margaret Thatcher came to power she considered privatising the NHS but pragmatically concluded that the NHS was too popular with the public to be disbanded (Timmins, 2017). Instead, she kept very tight control over NHS spending and decided to introduce a series of reforms to make it more 'business like'. In 1983, she charged the director of Sainsbury's, Roy Griffiths, with reforming the NHS. He introduced 'general managers' to take overall charge of services and introduced new business methods including tighter budgeting and 'performance management'. We look at these ideas in more detail in the next chapter when we discuss managerialism. Griffiths also introduced compulsory competitive tendering of ancillary services leading to services, such as ward cleaning being outsourced to the private sector. After the Griffiths reforms, management costs more than doubled with an enormous rise in senior manager posts (Pollock, 2020).

THE 'WORKING FOR PATIENTS' REFORMS, 1989

The most revolutionary change to the NHS, also instigated by Margaret Thatcher, was designed to further instill commercial principles into the service. In 1989, the 'Working for Patients' reforms introduced the **'internal market'** into the NHS. This would not be a real market but one that was politically controlled. For example, 'tariffs' for treatments were set by the government. Hospital and community services were to be run by self-governing 'trusts' under the control of a corporate board. A **'purchasing'** authority would buy services from these **'provider'** trusts under budgetary rules set out by the government. This new **'purchaser–provider split'** created an extra management tier that needed to be staffed and financed. Trusts were expected to compete with each other and with other providers in the private and voluntary sector through an elaborate annual contracting process (Webster, 2002). Some GP practices were allowed to become 'fundholders' who could also contract services. The new market was supposed to stimulate competition and its supporters argued that this would reduce costs and drive up efficiency. However, the internal market greatly increased management costs. It was also supposed to allow more consumer choice but, in practice, the internal market reduced patient choice, since it was the 'purchasing' agencies who decided where patients could go (Paton, 2016).

In the 1990s, the Major government became worried about the internal market reforms destabilising the service. Thus, the Department of Health held tight control over the service and contracts largely remained with existing providers (Timmins, 2017). However 'Working for Patients' had introduced a more financially driven ethos into the service, new layers of management and a cumbersome costing and contracting process. Nurses began to complain of the negative impact of market reforms on nursing culture (Traynor, 2012).

BLAIR AND 'NEW LABOUR' REFORMS

Tony Blair's Labour government inherited a service that was in severe financial difficulties but initially stuck to the previous government's spending plans. Blair remained committed to the market reforms instigated by Thatcher and, although 'purchasing' was renamed 'commissioning', the process was similar. The Blair government reorganised NHS structures several times. Commissioning was moved to Primary Care Groups which then became Primary Care Trusts. The government initially abolished fundholding but later introduced practice-based commissioning which was similar. It introduced a new tier of Strategic Health Authorities to oversee commissioning bodies and provider trusts. Hospital Trusts were renamed Foundation Trusts and given more financial independence (Paton, 2016).

Blair's government attempted to exercise greater control over the service and drive up standards while retaining the internal market. Two new regulators, the Care Quality Commission and the National Institute for Clinical Excellence were introduced. The government also introduced multiple performance targets creating what came to be described as a 'targets and terror' regime. In his second term of office, Blair increased NHS spending to match the European average. After this, there was a significant improvement in waiting times. It has since been debated as to whether the targets regime, as opposed to better funding, improved NHS performance (Edwards, 2021). Paton (2016) has argued that many opportunities for improving clinical services were missed because Blair wasted money needed for services on repeated management reorganisation.

CAMERON AND THE 2012 HEALTH AND SOCIAL CARE ACT

The 2010, Cameron government introduced the 2012 Health and Social Care Act sponsored by health minister, Andrew Lansley. Due to devolution, this Act only applied to England. This was yet another major reorganisation of the NHS occurring during a time of austerity when NHS spending again lagged behind the European average. The Act aimed to further 'marketise' the NHS and open up more NHS contracts to the private sector by allowing 'any qualified provider' to deliver NHS care. Outsourcing to the private sector steadily increased between 2013 and 2020 (Goodair & Reeves, 2022). The Act was strongly opposed by many sections of the public and was heavily amended during its passage through parliament (Timmins, 2017). A key objection was that the Act abolished the duty on the Secretary of State for Health to ensure that universal and comprehensive NHS services are available to all. This duty had existed since 1946 (Lister, 2012).

The reforms restructured the NHS by abolishing Primary Care Trusts and replacing them with 211 Clinical Commissioning Groups (CCG). CCGs were designed to further engage clinicians, such as GPs, in commissioning. The Act also abolished Strategic Health Authorities and replaced them with a single central body, NHS England, to oversee commissioning through the NHS Commissioning Board. The NHS was to be managed at a distance by NHS England. This was an 'arm's length' body, separate from the Department of Health with devolved powers. Its creation therefore weakened the democratic accountability of the NHS.

A central body called Public Health England was also set up to 'drive improvements' in public health. Local responsibility for public health was transferred from the NHS to new local authority 'Health and Wellbeing Boards' (HWBs). They have been described as being 'little more than talking shops' (Martin, 2020). The weakness and unaccountability of these new public health structures was exposed by their poor performance during the COVID-19 pandemic (Vize, 2020). The 2012 Act put additional strain on both NHS staff and NHS finances. These reforms applied in England but not to the devolved nations.

It is difficult to identify the true overall costs of this 'continuous revolution' of managerial and organisational changes over the last 40 years but they have been substantial. For example, in 2014, the government spent £640 million on management consultants to implement the 2012 Act (Kirkpatrick et al., 2019). There is no evidence that introduction of 'commissioning' has had any positive impact on the quality of services (Alderwick et al., 2021). Thus, repeated NHS reorganisations have absorbed enormous amounts of money, resources and staff energies and there has been little or no evidence that they have generated any improvement in the service. Despite lip service being paid to 'patient involvement', successive reorganisations have also steadily eroded democratic accountability and public involvement in the NHS.

The 2012 Act had fragmented the service and the damaging effects of this were exposed during the COVID-19 pandemic as the UK had one of the highest mortality rates among developed countries (Lawrence et al., 2020). According to Boyle et al. (2023), countries which had enacted neoliberal health reforms, such as the UK, had severely weakened public health provision and this meant that their populations were hit hardest by COVID-19. Nevertheless, in 2022 the government passed the Health and Care Act reorganising the NHS in England yet again.

JOHNSON AND THE HEALTH AND CARE ACT 2022

The Health and Care Act was passed in April 2022 under the Boris Johnson government. After the 2012 Act, NHS England began to pilot bodies called 'sustainability and transformation partnerships' (STPs) under a plan called the 'Five Year Forward View' (NHS England, 2015). The aims were said to be to address the fragmentation of the service caused by the 2012 Act and to control NHS costs. STPs were based on Accountable Care Organisations developed in the US but had no statutory authority. The purpose of the Five Year Forward View was stated as being to better integrate and coordinate local services and control costs (NHS England, 2015). Concerns were raised about the unaccountability of these new bodies which set about 'reconfiguring' services and also closed down some services (Pollock & Roderick, 2018). The Health and Care Act 2022 codified and extended the reforms trialled as a result of the Five Year Forward View and put them on a statutory footing. As a result, it has created the following new structures.

National Structures

NHS England now oversees and regulates the NHS. It incorporates a number of other agencies, such as NHS Improvement and NHS Digital. Public Health England has been split into the **UK Health Security Agency** and the **Office for Health Improvement and Disparities.** Both of these agencies now sit outside NHS England under the Department of Health and Social Care. It is unclear whether this move will improve the public health function or fragment it further (Paton, 2022). At a local level, public health remains with the 'Health and Wellbeing Boards' of local authorities despite their proven weaknesses (Hunter, 2020). The Act has not restored the duty on the Secretary of State to provide a universal and comprehensive health service. Instead, the **Department of Health and Social Care** will issue an **annual 'mandate'** to NHS England laying out its budget and its objectives for the year. There are thus concerns that the 2022 Act further undermines the universality of the service (Roderick & Pollock, 2022).

Integrated Care Boards (ICBs)

These will hold the budget for their area and be charged with the local planning, commissioning and oversight of NHS services. While the Act removes the purchaser–provider split, the 'integrated care system' must still engage in 'strategic commissioning' (Alderwick et al., 2021). ICBs replace Clinical Commissioning Groups and each cover roughly five times as many patients. There are 42 integrated care boards covering between half a million and 3 million people and an area the same size or larger than an English county; for example, NHS Greater Manchester, NHS Herefordshire and Worcestershire (Health Foundation, 2023). Critics have argued that these areas are far too large for integration to occur in a way that is meaningful at a clinical level (Paton, 2022).

ICBs contain a chair, chief executive, medical director, nursing director, finance director, two non-executive members and three 'partner members' nominated from NHS Trusts, primary care or local authorities. There is no patient or public representation. Due to their size, ICBs may be dealing with as many as 10 Trusts and 13 local authorities, so some provider organisations have no representation. Thus, there is a danger that ICBs could be dominated by a few powerful Trusts (Health Foundation, 2023). Although the new system promotes 'integration', controls over the contracting out of services to the private sector have been loosened. Some critics fear that the Act is intended to promote a more marketised system with mixed public and private provision and that this could lead to fragmentation, not integration (Roderick & Pollock, 2022).

Integrated Care Partnerships

Integrated care partnerships work with ICBs in an **'integrated care system'**. Integrated Care Partnerships (ICPs) are statutory committees bringing together the ICB and all the local authorities in the ICB's area. ICPs have a wider remit to look at the public health of the population.

Place-Based Partnerships

At a more local level it is envisaged that **'Place-Based Partnerships'** bring together NHS staff, local authorities, voluntary organisations and other 'community partners' to lead the design of integrated services in their areas (King's Fund, 2022). It is at this level that the integration of health and social care might be addressed. It remains to be seen how this might or might not work out in practice as 'partnership working' in health and social care does not have a successful history (Martin, 2020). At a neighbourhood level, the Act also envisaged that **'primary care networks'** of GPs, pharmacists, dentists and opticians should work together to coordinate services.

The new Act introduced an enormously complex structure at a time when the NHS was under great strain in the aftermath of COVID-19. The NHS faced a huge backlog of demand, further 'efficiency' savings and industrial unrest from staff exhausted by the pandemic. According to Hartley (2023), the NHS was still 'fire fighting' so had little chance to get to grips with the new structures. This was compounded by a lack of clarity about the role of ICBs and about the roles and responsibilities of every tier in the new structure. There is also little evidence that the new structures will solve the problems in social care (Alderwick et al., 2021).

Other key concerns about the new structure are that it will undermine the NHS as a universal service, since NHS England is not required to provide a comprehensive service (Roderick & Pollock, 2022). This new system could end up recreating the same 'patchwork' of services as existed before the NHS. The new system lacks democratic accountability and there is little evidence of patient and public involvement in the new structures. Roderick and Pollock also suggest that the Act also allows more 'corporate penetration' of the NHS by allowing 200 'accredited' private companies, such as management consultancies into every level of NHS administration. Past reorganisations of the NHS have provided few benefits but many negative effects (Alderwick et al., 2021). It is difficult to imagine that this latest reorganisation will be any different.

Key Policy Issues

DEVOLUTION

Since 1999, the NHS in Scotland, Wales and Northern Ireland has been organised separately by the devolved governments. Neither the 2012 Act nor the 2022 Act have applied to the devolved nations. However, the UK government still controls the spending that it allocates to the devolved nations so the devolved nations lack full control over their health spending. In the case of Wales, funding has been poorer than other areas of the UK (Paton, 2022). All three nations have been moving away, to varying degrees, from the market reforms that continue to be pursued in England. The devolved nations have also diverged in other ways. Wales has put a particular focus on integration and developing community care. Both Scotland and Wales have abolished the internal market and returned to directly managed services. Scotland has also introduced free personal care for the elderly and increased spending on social care (Timmins, 2017). Prescriptions are now free in Scotland, Wales and Northern Ireland but not in England.

FUNDING AND COST CONTROL

We noted when discussing the origin of the NHS that, from the start, critics have suggested that it was too expensive, wasteful and inefficient. These objections are usually raised by those who are politically opposed to a universal, publicly funded and owned service. Edwards (2022) argues that they are a myth. A directly managed service funded by taxation has the advantage of simplicity and very low administrative costs, so in the first few decades of the NHS, administrative costs were very low. However, since 1989, this advantage has been undermined by repeated reforms which have increased the administrative complexity of the service; increased management costs and reduced the proportion of NHS funding that could be spent on clinical care (Paton, 2016). In addition, when we compare the UK to its European neighbours, it has also consistently spent less on healthcare. In 2019, the UK spent 18% less on healthcare than the European average (Health Foundation, 2022). Greener (2018) has argued that it is increased spending, not managerial reform, that improves NHS services.

However, since the 1980s, the NHS has been subject to year-on-year efficiency drives, in order to obtain 'more for less' from the service and NHS reforms have mainly been focused on this drive for greater efficiency rather than other issues, such as patient choice or care quality. Typically, NHS institutions are set a target figure of 'efficiency savings' that services must find from within their budgets. Management consultancy firms, such as McKinsey and Company, have often been paid to find these 'efficiencies' (Bogdanich & Forsythe, 2023). However, Kirkpatrick et al. (2019) have shown that the use of management consultants increases inefficiencies. These 'efficiencies' have become progressively more difficult to find as these demands are repeated year on year. Thus, under the Cameron government's austerity programme the Treasury demanded £20 billion in 'efficiency savings' in an exercise called the 'Nicholson challenge' (Paton, 2016). The government's 'mandate' to the NHS in 2023 included 'cash releasing efficiency savings' of 2.2% in 2023–2024. Thus, with a backlog of unmet needs post COVID-19, the NHS again faced real-term spending cuts (Pope, 2023).

The pressure to cut the costs of care has been continuous leading to reductions in the length of hospital stays, reduced staffing levels, skill mix dilution and closures of services. In 1979, the NHS had 361,670 hospital beds but had lost 120,000 of these by 1992 due to cuts and hospital closures under Thatcher (Hansard, 1993). By 2019, the NHS had lost roughly 100,000 more, leaving just 141,000 beds, with an increased proportion of these being 'day' beds (King's Fund, 2021). Thus, during a 40-year period of NHS 'reform', the service has lost almost two-thirds of its hospital beds. While other countries have also cut hospital beds, the UK is an outlier in terms of the severity of its cuts. The average number of beds per 1000 people is 5 in other European countries but the figure for the UK is less than half this at 2.4. Germany, by contrast, has 7.8 (BMA, 2022). Jones (2023) suggests that healthcare in England is 'sliding into chaos' due to the savagery of its cuts in hospital beds.

RATIONING CARE

Funding constraints means that services are rationed; some needs are not met or care is delayed. Much rationing is implicit; for example, clinical staff have to prioritise care and some patients have to wait. Missed and unfinished nursing care due to heavy workloads can also be seen as a form of implicit rationing which can have a negative effect on patient outcomes (Schubert et al., 2012).

In the UK, there has been increased use of more explicit rationing. The National Institute for Health and Care Excellence appraises treatments and decides which should be provided by the NHS. It also produces clinical guidelines outlining what it considers the optimal evidence-based treatment regime for specific health problems. England and Wales follow NICE guidance whereas Scotland is more selective in its implementation of NICE guidelines. NICE is required to take into account both the effectiveness of treatments and their value for money and thus acts as a rationing body. It uses a measure called QALY (Quality Adjusted Life Years) to appraise the value of a treatment.

A QALY is seen as equivalent to 1 year of perfect health while death is rated at zero. Living with a disability or illness for 1 year will be 'quality adjusted' to a figure that is less than one, so, for example, a person with a chronic illness may be rated as having a QALY of just 0.75 (McCabe, 2009) The use of this measure raises serious ethical questions about how we value life and, in particular, the lives of people with disabilities. This is a particularly important ethical issue when the QALY is used to evaluate lifesaving treatments. It has been suggested that disability discrimination has been embedded in this measure which rates the disabled as of lesser value than the able bodied (John et al., 2017). Mulkay et al. (1987) have also suggested that the QALY has a very narrow view of how to value human life, prioritising an economic view and excluding other value systems.

PERFORMANCE MANAGEMENT AND REGULATION

The 1989 reforms which introduced the 'internal market' ended the clear lines of accountability that had previously existed in the NHS. A directly managed service had been replaced with 'self-governing' providers who had a contractual relationship with 'purchasing' authorities. It had been argued that the reforms would 'free' hospitals to be more autonomous but the reality was very different. Paradoxically, the new system would result in a blizzard of new centrally set rules, regulations and targets, devised by the Department of Health, to enable the government to keep control of the service (Timmins, 2017).

In addition, a number of new regulatory agencies would be set up to oversee the service. In particular, the Care Quality Commission (CQC) was set up under the Blair government to regulate standards of quality and safety in health and social care settings. The CQC regularly monitors and inspects services and rates them on a five-point scale from outstanding to inadequate. Sanctions are taken against services which 'require improvement' or are 'inadequate' to ensure failings are addressed. These changes have been described as the rise of the 'regulatory state'. Privatisation and 'marketisation' of services has led to a growth of regulatory activity and regulatory bodies to replace the 'command and control' systems that exist in directly managed state services. Market systems are supposed to reduce 'bureaucracy' but, ironically, this new 'regulatory' form of bureaucracy has sharply increased bureaucratic work. This has particularly increased the burden of paperwork on frontline staff. We will look more at this new form of bureaucracy in the next chapter.

REFLECTION POINT

Think about your own experience of the NHS. What do you think are the most important policy issues facing the service? How do you think these should be addressed? What evidence could you draw on to support your arguments?

Summary of Key Points

- Policymaking is only partially influenced by evidence. Political factors, the media and 'policy entrepreneurs' all influence the policy process.

- Two main political philosophies (social democracy and neoliberalism) have influenced UK health policy. While social democracy shaped the creation of the NHS, neoliberalism has dominated recent health policies, particularly in England.
- In the last 40 years, there has been a 'continuous revolution' in the NHS with repeated reorganisations of the service. Evidence suggests this has been detrimental to the service.
- Spending on UK healthcare has been tightly constrained over many years and has fallen behind spending in comparable nations.

Further Reading

Calnan, M. (2020). *Health policy, power and politics: Sociological insights*. Emerald Publishing Limited.

Garland, D (2016). *The welfare state: A very short introduction*. Oxford University Press.

Smith, H. L. (2014). *Harry's last stand: How the world my generation built is falling down, and what we can do to save it*. Icon Books Ltd.

References

Alderwick, H., Dunn, P., Gardner, T., Mays, N., & Dixon, J. (2021). Will a new NHS structure in England help recovery from the pandemic? *BMJ, 372*, 1–5.

BMA. (2022). *NHS hospital beds data analysis*. Retrieved February 1, 2024, from https://www.bma.org.uk/advice-and-support/nhs-delivery-and-workforce/pressures/nhs-hospital-beds-data-analysis.

Bogdanich, W., & Forsythe, M. (2023). *When McKinsey comes to town: The hidden influence of the world's most powerful consulting firm*. Penguin Books.

Bovis, J. L., Edwin, J. P., Bano, C. P., Tyraskis, A., Baskaran, D., & Karuppaiah, K. (2018). Barriers to staff reporting adverse incidents in NHS hospitals. *Future Healthcare Journal, 5*(2), 117.

Boyle, M., Hickson, J., & Gomez, K. U. (2023). *COVID-19 and the case against neoliberalism: The United Kingdom's political pandemic*. Springer.

Cairney, P. (2019). *Understanding public policy: Theories and issues*. Bloomsbury Publishing.

Cairney, P. (2021). The UK government's COVID-19 policy: What does "guided by the science" mean in practice? *Frontiers in Political Science, 3*, 624068.

Calnan, M. (2020). *Health policy, power and politics: Sociological insights*. Emerald Publishing Limited.

Cohen, S. (2020). *The NHS: Britain's National Health Service* (pp. 1948–2020). Bloomsbury Publishing.

Colebatch, H. (2009). *Policy*. McGraw-Hill Education.

Davies, P. (2012). Behind closed doors: How much power does McKinsey wield? *BMJ, 344*, e2905.

Department of Health and Social Care (DHSC). (2022). *Women's health strategy for England*. Retrieved December 6, 2023, from https://www.gov.uk/government/publications/womens-health-strategy-for-england/womens-health-strategy-for-england.

Edwards, N. (2021). Turning up the heat on the NHS. *BMJ, 375*, n2618.

Edwards N (2022). 'Myth #1: "We already spend too much on health—and despite this our outcomes are poor"'. Nuffield Trust blog, 19 October. Retrieved February 1, 2024, from https://www.nuffieldtrust.org.uk/news-item/myth-1-we-already-spend-too-much-on-health-and-our-outcomes-are-poor.

Garland, D. (2016). *The welfare state: A very short introduction*. Oxford University Press.

Goodair, B., & Reeves, A. (2022). Outsourcing health-care services to the private sector and treatable mortality rates in England, 2013–20: An observational study of NHS privatisation. *The Lancet Public Health, 7*(7), e638–e646.

Goode, E., & Ben-Yehuda, N. (2010). *Moral panics: The social construction of deviance*. John Wiley & Sons.

Greener, I. (2018). Learning from New Labour's approach to the NHS. *Social Policy Review, 30*, 249–268.

Hansard. (1993). *NHS beds*. (Vol. 223), April 20th. Retrieved February 1, 2024, from https://hansard.parliament.uk/Commons/1993-04-20/debates/773c0bf9-b1ab-4bac-96e3-cfefcefae6ee/NhsBeds.

Harrison, S., & Wood, B. (1999). Designing health service organization in the UK, 1968 to 1998: From blueprint to bright idea and 'manipulated emergence'. *Public Administration, 77*(4), 751–768.

Hartley. (2023). Year one of integrated care systems has been tough—here's what they need in year two. *NHS Providers Blog*. 30th June. Retrieved February 1, 2024, from https://nhsproviders.org/news-blogs/blogs/year-one-of-integrated-care-systems-has-been-tough-heres-what-they-need-in-year-two.

Hastings, G. (2012). Why corporate power is a public health priority. *BMJ, 345*, e5124.

Hayek, F. A. (2009). *The road to serfdom: Text and documents—The definitive edition*. University of Chicago Press.

Health Foundation. (2022). *How does UK health spending compare across Europe over the past decade?* https://www.health.org.uk/news-and-comment/charts-and-infographics/how-does-uk-health-spending-compare-across-europe-over-the-past-decade.

Health Foundation. (2023). *Integrated care boards: What do they look like?* https://www.health.org.uk/news-and-comment/blogs/integrated-care-boards-what-do-they-look-like.

Herbert, S. M. (1939). *Britain's Health*. Penguin Books.

Hewison, A., & Griffiths, M. (2004). Leadership development in health care: A word of caution. *Journal of Health Organization and Management, 18*(6), 464–473.

Hoefer, R. (2022). The multiple streams framework: Understanding and applying the problems, policies, and politics approach. *Journal of Policy Practice and Research, 3*(1), 1–5.

Hope, D., & Limberg, J. (2020). *The economic consequences of major tax cuts for the rich*. International Inequalities Institute Working Papers (55), London School of Economics and Political Science.

Hunter, D. J. (2020). Strictly come partnering: Are health and wellbeing boards the answer? In A. Bonner (Ed.), *Local authorities and the social determinants of health* (pp. 67–82). Policy Press.

John, T. M., Millum, J., & Wasserman, D. (2017). How to allocate scarce health resources without discriminating against people with disabilities. *Economics & Philosophy, 33*(2), 161–186.

Jones, R. P. (2023). Addressing the knowledge deficit in hospital bed planning and defining an optimum region for the number of different types of hospital beds in an effective health care system. *International Journal of Environmental Research and Public Health, 20*(24), 7171.

King's Fund. (2021). *NHS hospital bed numbers: Past, present, future*. Retrieved February 1, 2024, from https://www.kingsfund.org.uk/publications/nhs-hospital-bed-numbers?gclid=CjwKCAjwgsqoBhBNEiwAwe5w08M6lSgAEq1O57qkHN-wbOWEzVLxxZ4A3Gds05N7zMOeuk7T9xuSbhoCCWYQAvD_BwE.

King's Fund. (2022). *Integrated care systems: How will they work under the Health and Care Act?* Retrieved February 1, 2024, from https://www.kingsfund.org.uk/insight-and-analysis/data-and-charts/integrated-care-systems-health-and-care-act#integrated-care-systems.

Kingdon, J. W. (1993). How do issues get on public policy agendas? In Wilson, W. J. (Ed.), *Sociology and the public agenda* (pp. 40–53). Sage Publications.

Kirkpatrick, I., Sturdy, A. J., Alvarado, N., Blanco-Oliver, A., & Veronesi, G. (2019). 'The impact of management consultants on public service efficiency'. *Policy & Politics, 47*(1), 77–95.

Kynaston, D. (2008). *Austerity Britain* (pp. 1945–1951). A&C Black. (Vol. 1).

Lawrence, F., Garside, J., Pegg, D., Conn, D., Carell, S., & Davies, H. (2020). *How a decade of privatization and cuts exposed England to coronavirus*. The Guardian 31st May.

Levitt, R. (1976). *The reorganised National Health Service*. Croom Helm Ltd.

Lister, J. (2005). *Health policy reform: Driving the wrong way? A critical guide to the global 'health reform' industry*. Middlesex University Press.

Lister, J. (2012). In defiance of the evidence: Conservatives threaten to 'reform' away England's National Health Service. *International Journal of Health Services, 42*(1), 137–155.

Looi, J. C., & Kisely, S. R. (2019). Potemkin redux: The re-disorganisation of public mental health services in Australia. *Australasian Psychiatry, 27*(6), 607–610.

Mahajan, R. P. (2010). Critical incident reporting and learning. *British Journal of Anaesthesia, 105*(1), 69–75.

Mannion, R., & Small, N. (2019). On folk devils, moral panics and new wave public health. *International Journal of Health Policy and Management, 8*(12), 678–683.

Martin, G. (2020). Partnership and accountability in the era of integrated care: A tale from England. *Journal of Health Services Research & Policy, 25*(1), 1–3.

Maynard, A., & Bloor, K. (1998). *Managed care: Panacea or palliation*. The Nuffield Trust.

McCabe, C. (2009). *What is cost-utility analysis*. Retrieved September 12, 2023, from http://www.bandolier.org.uk/painres/download/whatis/What_is_cost-util.pdf.

Ministry of Health. (1944). *A National Health Service*. HMSO Cmd. 6502.

Ministry of Health. (1956). *Report of the committee of inquiry into the cost of the NHS (Guillebaud Inquiry)*. HMSO Cmd. 9663.

Mulkay, M., Ashmore, M., & Pinch, T. (1987). Measuring the quality of life: A sociological intervention concerning the application of economics to health care. *Sociology, 21*(4), 541–564.

National Archives. (2017). *The beveridge report and the foundations of the welfare state*. Retrieved February 1, 2024, from https://blog.nationalarchives.gov.uk/beveridge-report-foundations-welfare-state/.

NHS England. (2015). *Five year forward view*. Retrieved February 1, 2024, from https://www.england.nhs.uk/wp-content/uploads/2015/06/5yfv-time-to-deliver-25-06.pdf.

Orgad, S., & Rottenberg, C. (2023). The menopause moment: The rising visibility of 'the change' in UK news coverage. *European Journal of Cultural Studies*, 13675494231159562.

Paton, C. (2016). *The politics of health policy reform in the UK: England's permanent revolution*. Springer.

Paton, C. (2022). *NHS reform and health politics in the UK: Revolution, counter-revolution and Covid crisis*. Springer.

Paton, C. (2023). The NHS in the UK at 75: On life support or death watch? It's the politics, stupid (to misquote Bill Clinton). *The International Journal of Health Planning and Management, 38*(6), 1601–1612.

Pollock, A. M., & Roderick, P. (2018). Why we should be concerned about accountable care organisations in England's NHS. *BMJ, 360*, k364.

Pollock, A. M. (2020). *NHS plc: The privatisation of our health care*. Verso Books.

Pope, C. (2023). NHS waiting times: A government pledge. *BMJ, 380*, 71.

Roderick, P., & Pollock, A. M. (2022). Dismantling the National Health Service in England. *International Journal of Health Services, 52*(4), 470–479.

Sayer, A. (2014). *Why we can't afford the rich*. Policy Press.

Schubert, M., Clarke, S. P., Aiken, L. H., & De Geest, S. (2012). Associations between rationing of nursing care and inpatient mortality in Swiss hospitals. *International Journal for Quality in Health Care, 24*(3), 230–238.

Seear, K. (2016). *The makings of a modern epidemic: Endometriosis, gender and politics*. Routledge.

Smith, A. (2008). An inquiry into the nature and causes of the wealth of nations. In Biggart, N. W. (Ed.), *Readings in economic sociology* (pp. 1–17). John Wiley & Sons.

Smith, H. L. (2014). *Harry's last stand: How the world my generation built is falling down, and what we can do to save it*. Icon Books Ltd.

Sridhar, D. (2023). Ignore the Johnson and Sunak circus: These are the real lessons from the Covid inquiry. *The Guardian Weekly*. https://www.theguardian.com/commentisfree/2023/dec/12/political-blame-game-covid-inquiry-pandemic.

Steger, M. B., & Roy, R. K. (2010). *Neoliberalism: A very short introduction*. Oxford University Press.

Tawney, R. H. (1952). *Equality*. Allen.

Timmins, N. (2017). *The five giants: A biography of the welfare state*. William Collins.

Traynor, M. (2012). *Managerialism and nursing: Beyond oppression and profession*. Routledge.

Traynor, M. (2013). *Nursing in context: Policy, politics, profession*. Bloomsbury Publishing.

UN General Assembly. (1948). *Universal declaration of human rights*. UN General Assembly.

Vize, R. (2020). How the erosion of our public health system hobbled England's Covid-19 response. *BMJ, 369*, m1934.

Webster, C. (2002). *The National Health Service: A political history*. Oxford University Press.

CHAPTER 9

Professionalism, Managerialism and Nursing Work

Introduction

This chapter briefly considers the history of professions before looking at the changing nature of professionalism in the twenty-first century. It examines the reasons for the changes to professional roles and occupational boundaries in healthcare. It considers the growing influence of managerialism and its impact on professional autonomy. The chapter also examines changes in professional boundaries and the creation of new 'hybrid' occupations, such as the physician associate. It reviews debates about the status and value of professionalism and its future. The second part of the chapter looks at the history and development of nursing; nursing as 'women's work'; the nature of nursing work and the impact of managerialism on nursing work.

WHAT IS PROFESSIONALISM?

The term 'profession' comes from the Latin word 'professus' which means to make a vow of allegiance. It described dedication to a knowledge-based discipline. We can date this idea of professionalism back to the Greek physician, Hippocrates, and his formulation of the Hippocratic Oath in 400 BC (Smith, 1996). The earliest professions were law, medicine and divinity, taught from the Middle Ages onward. As medicine in the UK developed as a profession, it became organised in a way that separated it from other healing occupations, such as apothecaries, particularly through the creation of medical Royal Colleges. This gave doctors an elite status and more control over the domain of healing. This led, eventually, to medicine becoming a state-registered profession in 1858 (Lawrence, 2006). Midwifery became a state-registered profession in 1902, followed by nursing in 1919. State registration gave these occupations a protected status. This prohibited other occupations from using their titles and, to some extent, from encroaching on their territory. It also granted them a degree of independence through self-regulation (Hallett & Cooke, 2011).

Professions are knowledge-based occupations which provide a service. An early, influential attempt to define professions was Flexner's **'trait approach'**. In 1915, Flexner said that a profession had to have a number of key 'traits', such as exercising **individual responsibility**, being **based in learning**, having **specialised skills**, being **self-organising** and being **altruistic** (Flexner, 2001). Flexner thought occupations such as nursing and social work would never be truly autonomous professions. Instead, he saw them as subordinate 'arms' of medicine. Flexner made a sharp distinction between professionalism and commercialism, seeing risks to the public good from the latter's narrow pursuit of profit (Hafferty & Castellani, 2010). Following Flexner, other authors added new attributes. Thus, according to Greenwood (1957), professions should also have a **code of ethics, be regulated by the state**, and entry should be governed by a **formal examination of competence**.

The trait approach suggested that professionals should be granted some autonomy and in return they would uphold high ethical standards and practice lifelong dedication to the art and science of their profession. This was considered important in order for professionals to inspire the trust of their clients and patients. In 1958, the sociologist Emile Durkheim wrote that the professions were socially important institutions which acted as **'moral communities'** (Durkheim, 2013). He thought they played a vital role in society by promoting what he called **'civic morals'** such as altruism and public service. Durkheim thought these ethics were maintained through a collegial culture but could be undermined by political and commercial interests.

By contrast, later authors took a much more cynical and pessimistic view of the professions and cast doubt on the ethical claims of professional groups. These critics rejected the idea of professional altruism, instead seeing professions as self-interested groups who wielded too much power. Reality, they said, rarely lived up to the ideals that the professions claimed to follow (Johnson, 2016). Reasons for this cynicism towards professions, particularly medicine, were varied. Firstly, individual cases of patient or client abuse had undermined trust in the professions; secondly, the disability rights movement had rightly criticised the ways in which professionals held power over disabled people's lives. Finally, the growing consumer movement, which championed consumer choice, also began to target professions such as medicine. The growth of consumerism was itself linked to the growing influence of neoliberal ideas which saw the market as the best instrument for regulating public services and distrusted public service values. This, in turn, was linked to the rise of managerialism which also challenged the power and autonomy of professionals (Steger & Roy, 2010). Thus, the critics of professionalism had quite varied, and sometimes conflicting, motives and values.

For the critics of professionalism, the only distinguishing features of professions worth noting were their power and autonomy. Drawing on the ideas of the sociologist, Max Weber (Gerth & Mills, 2014), they saw the one key characteristic of the professions as **'professional closure'** (Larson, 2012). Weber had described 'social closure' as the process through which occupational groups gain monopoly control over a field of practice in order to improve their economic position and status. From this more cynical point of view all the trappings of professionalism, such as the long period of education, professional registration and a code of ethics, served no purpose apart from protecting the power and status of the group (Porter, 1998). Crompton (1990) disagreed with this negative analysis of the professions arguing that, like all occupations, professions try to protect their livelihoods but they can at the same time be altruistic. She said these contradictions were found in many other public service occupations, such as firefighting.

A key critic of professionalism (and of the medical profession) was Freidson (1988) who said that professions were distinguished from other occupations by their **professional dominance** over a particular area of work. He believed that traditional professions, particularly medicine, had gained too much power. Medicine, he said, had engaged in **'medical imperialism'** gaining authority over more and more areas of our lives (see the discussion of medicalisation in Chapter 6). In later work, Freidson (2001) qualified his criticisms of the professions. He returned to Durkheim's idea of 'civic values' describing professionalism as a **'third logic'** which could offer an alternative to commercial and bureaucratic values. He said, however, that if professionalism was to be rescued as a force for good it needed to modernise. Professionals needed to become more open and work in partnership with patients. He thought that health professions still had an important role to play in defending both patients' interests and the quality of services (Freidson, 2001). Many professional groups have since attempted to foster these ideas by encouraging transparency, patient partnerships and service user involvement.

Despite traditional professions being under attack in the late twentieth century, many other occupations were striving to attain professional status. Usually, this was through a **'credentialist'** approach. Credentialism involves trying to raise the status of an occupation by raising the level of qualifications needed to enter it, such as raising nursing qualifications to degree level. Since these attempts to achieve professional status have coincided with the expansion of higher education, many occupations aspiring to professional status have found themselves competing to raise their qualifications to merely stand still. In the 1960s, only 4% of school leavers went into higher education, compared to over 40% today (Lightfoot, 2016). If educational qualifications are increasing across a wide range of occupations (e.g. degrees are now available in hairdressing and circus skills), then an occupation, such as nursing, cannot afford to fall behind, but will not necessarily raise its status. In 1964, Wilensky had described this as **'the professionalisation of everyone'**. He saw many modern occupations as characterised by a competitive striving for professional identity. He believed, however, that most would not manage to improve their status.

CHANGES TO PROFESSIONALISM

We have seen that professionalism has become a changing and contested idea. Freidson (2001) hoped for a new version of professionalism in which the professions embraced a spirit of openness, and worked collaboratively with patients and clients. By contrast, Evetts (2011) had a very different analysis of how what she calls the **'new professionalism'** has actually developed. She said that the key feature of modern professionals was that they work in large-scale organisations, whether commercial or state run, and are now subject to intensive technical and bureaucratic control. These new professionals are no longer trusted by their employers to exercise professional discretion but work in low-trust cultures where they are subject to higher levels of managerial scrutiny. In healthcare, this is often justified with reference to the need to deliver evidence-based practice (Saarni & Gylling, 2004). However, the drive to control professionals and standardise their work also has other motives, such as increasing managerial control and driving down costs (Germov, 2005). These new controls involve detailed performance management and measurement, strict cost controls and the standardisation of work through the use of protocols and procedures. The professions have also been 'restratified', creating a new management hierarchy within the professions. Professionals who have left the clinical field for management now wield power over their clinical colleagues. This has marked an end to professional collegiality (Freidson, 1983).

Healthcare organisations have also made attempts to break down the boundaries between the professions by introducing new 'hybrid' roles, such as physician associates who act as doctor substitutes (NHS England, 2017). These roles are justified on the grounds of workforce shortages and financial pressures. These 'hybrid' workers are often cheaper; have less autonomy than the medical professionals that they replace but, as yet, have no clear career pathways. Job titles, regulatory arrangements, support structures, educational preparation and lines of accountability for these roles are still inconsistent across organisations (Fothergill et al., 2022; Hooks & Walker, 2020). Noordegraaf (2007) has suggested that recent changes in how professions are managed, and how their role boundaries are defined, mean that professionalism is now a more ambiguous concept.

A more critical approach to the changes described above sees, instead of a 'new' professionalism, the **'deprofessionalisation'** of occupations. According to McKinlay and Stoeckle (2020) we are witnessing the **'proletarianisation'** of occupations such as medicine; in other words, their status and class position are being downgraded. They describe proletarianisation as the process through which occupations lose control over the content of their training and education; the tools and conditions of their work; their autonomy regarding the content of their work and what they are paid for their work. Thus, McKinlay and Marceau (2002) predict a decline in the pay, conditions and autonomy of professional groups. The recent industrial action over declining pay and conditions of work by health professions in the UK lends some support to their arguments (Abbasi, 2023). In addition, self-regulation has declined with the regulation of the professions increasingly coming under state control. For example, the Nursing and Midwifery Council (NMC) founded in 2002 is wholly appointed by the government, whereas its predecessor contained clinical nurses elected by the profession. Although the NMC contains some nursing registrants, these are not clinical nurses; its members almost exclusively come from managerial backgrounds (UK Government, 2011).

Other critics of deprofessionalisation have highlighted the negative effects for clients and patients of **'captive professionals'** who are ethically and professionally compromised by the pressures of the organisation that employs them. Captive professionals act as agents of that organisation rather than acting in the client's interest and can no longer exercise professional discretion. This may entail refusing or rationing services or exercising social control functions on behalf of an organisation or the state (Freund et al., 2003). For example, we saw in Chapter 4 how health professionals have been required to administer immigration controls as part of the 'hostile environment' policy. Another example is healthcare professionals who assess 'work capability' on behalf of the Department of Work and Pensions and are under pressure to meet its targets (McCartney, 2011).

PROFESSIONAL DISCRETION AND CLINICAL JUDGEMENT

Evetts' (2011) description of 'new' professionalism is of workers who follow protocols and procedures and have little **professional discretion**. When we talk about professional discretion we mean that health professionals have the freedom to assess individual cases and some freedom to exercise their professional judgement, taking into account a range of factors including both the unique circumstances of the patient and situational or organisational constraints (Cheraghi-Sohi & Calnan, 2013). The use of professional discretion does not preclude the use of evidence-based guidelines but allows flexibility in modifying these to fit a particular situation or individual patient.

An analysis of the nature of professional discretion by two medical historians suggested that it could be understood by looking at two key components of knowledge-based occupations (Jamous & Pelloille, 1970). They called these two components **'indeterminacy'** and **'technicality'**.

- **Technicality** refers to cases or situations which are clear-cut and unambiguous and which can therefore be covered by a set of technical rules, protocols and procedures. For example, engineers may be able to assess with mathematical accuracy the load-bearing capacity of a structure and this can then be governed by technical rules.
- **Indeterminacy** means something (a case or situation) that is uncertain and ambiguous. Thus, it cannot be easily defined and measured and, as a result, it cannot be subject to a fixed set of rules. In professional work it refers to cases or situations that require the judgement of highly experienced and knowledgeable experts. In healthcare, professionals link the idea of indeterminacy to the importance of building a relationship with patients and knowing patients as individuals rather than cases; this allows each patient to be treated as a unique case and their care to be personalised. This is particularly important when individuals' have complex health problems (Hughes et al., 2008).

Indeterminate situations may require the use of what Polanyi (1958) has called **'tacit'** knowledge as opposed to **'explicit'** knowledge. By tacit knowledge we mean knowledge that is gained by experience and is difficult to put into words; also sometimes called intuition. We can often only see it in action, for example, in the virtuoso musician. In healthcare, we see it where professionals are able to read complex situations intuitively based on experience; for example, the nurse who 'just knows' that a patient is 'not herself' ahead of any evidence of deterioration showing up on the early warning score. Studies have shown that tacit knowledge plays an important role in nurses' early detection of patient deterioration which cannot be fully replaced by the various early warning scores available (Odell et al., 2009).

The downsides of professional discretion can be, firstly, that some professionals may overestimate their knowledge and expertise and, secondly, that it can allow social biases to enter into treatment decisions as we have seen in our discussions of sexism in healthcare in Chapter 3. However, as we also saw in earlier chapters, social biases can also be found in protocols, guidelines and measures. The use of protocols can prevent poor care but this can sometimes be at the expense of downgrading excellent individualised care to average standardised care.

According to Jamous and Pelloille (1970) all occupations involve a mixture of technical and indeterminate knowledge. What varies between occupations is the amount of indeterminate knowledge needed and whether that indeterminate knowledge is recognised. This determines whether clinical judgement and professional discretion are allowed. In healthcare, the autonomy of doctors started to be undermined along with their freedom to exercise clinical judgement as a result of managerialism (see section on managerialism). Thus the 'new' professionalism described by Evetts (2011) marks the success of a managerialist project designed to significantly curtail the clinical freedom of expert professionals.

REFLECTION POINT

We have discussed the concept 'indeterminacy' or professional 'discretion'. How much of a role do you think that professional 'discretion' should play in contemporary healthcare? What are the advantages and disadvantages of limiting professional (clinical) judgement?

Managerialism in Healthcare

THE IDEA OF MANAGERIALISM

The term 'managerialism' has been used to describe a cascade of changes to public services from the 1980s onwards. Two things came together to produce these changes: firstly, changes in the occupational ambitions of management as a discipline, and secondly, the rise of neoliberalism (see Chapter 8). We will look at the more general idea of managerialism first and then consider the particular form that managerialism took in public services.

According to Klikauer (2015), managerialism arose as a result of a new ideology being promoted through US business schools from the mid-twentieth century. This ideology suggested that all organisations are essentially the same; there is no fundamental difference between a hospital, car factory, coal mine or university and all can be 'optimised' by the application of 'general management' skills. Managerialism thus claimed it had exclusive knowledge of how to run organisations. Business schools in the US promoted the idea that 'general managers' should hold leadership positions in all organisations, replacing and controlling local professional experts such as doctors, engineers and scientists (Klikauer, 2015). Klikauer is thus suggesting that managerialism is an imperialist project far more ambitious in scope than the 'medical imperialism' criticised by Freidson (1988).

The body of expertise promoted by managerialism leans heavily on what has been called **Taylorism**. In the early twentieth century, the mechanical engineer, Frederick Winslow Taylor, wanted to tighten controls over workers to increase their productivity. He described workers as 'economic animals' who should allow managers to think for them (Watson, 2017). He thought that work should be broken down into its smallest component tasks so these could be measured and timed. He timed workers with stopwatches in order to lay down tight procedures for carrying out tasks (called the 'one best way') so that managers could both speed workers up and also employ cheaper, less skilled workers. He also favoured what he called a 'minimum interaction' style of management, believing managers should control frontline workers remotely through rules, procedures and measuring systems. Taylor sometimes compared workers to draft animals, such as oxen (Taylor, 2004). Some critics of Taylorism have suggested that racism and the legacy of the US slave system were embedded into scientific management at its outset; through its conception of workers as animals who were there to be controlled and his adoption of some of the disciplinary practices of the slave system (Aufhauser, 1973; Cooke, 2003). In healthcare, Taylorism can be seen in the efforts to get 'more for less' from the workforce; where managers are remote; where workers are governed by procedures and paperwork and where production-line models of caregiving have been introduced (Wong, 2004).

Managerialism has since had global reach. As a result, authors have suggested that it is also culturally imperialist, allowing the US to impose its ideas about how public service organisations should be run on other cultures through international organisations such as the World Bank (Braddock et al., 2006). Managerialism also seeks to colonise the **'lifeworld'** (see Chapter 5), exporting its ideology of business efficiency into even the most personal aspects of our lives. We are now all supposed to 'project manage' our own lives and families (Sotirin et al., 2007) while patients are expected to 'self-manage' their illnesses (see Chapter 7). Piketty (2014) has argued that the growth of managerialism has also contributed to the widening social inequalities of contemporary capitalism. We saw this in the enormous increase in pay disparity between managers and their workforces described in Chapter 2.

NEOLIBERALISM AND NEW PUBLIC MANAGEMENT

Managerialism has taken a particular form in public services. This has been called 'new public management' (NPM). In NPM, we see two ideologies brought together, namely, neoliberalism and managerialism. As discussed in the previous chapter, neoliberalism refers to a belief in the 'free market' and in the idea that market principles should enter and control most areas of our lives, supplanting other values.

American management consultants started to lay out a set of prescriptions for the neoliberal reform of public services which came to be known as 'new public management' (Hood, 1991). Key principles of new public management included:

- Introducing competition between service providers by creating a 'managed market'
- Promoting consumerism by rating and ranking services
- A focus on service outputs rather than on resources in order to get 'more for less'
- Encouraging public services to generate income
- 'Empowering' service users by handing back responsibilities. For example, promoting 'self-management' (Osborne & Gaebler, 1993).

As we saw in Chapter 8, a new era of NPM in UK health service was introduced by the 'Griffths' reforms in the 1980s. These reforms put general managers in charge and introduced Taylorist management practices to exercise more control over health professionals. There was also a programme of neoliberal reform of public services, such as the education system and the NHS, involving repeated reorganisations to 'modernise' them in order to make them behave more like the private sector. Despite a rhetorical focus on choice and consumerism, the primary focus of NPM has been on cost efficiency and on curbing state spending. Simonet (2015) has argued that NPM has been a failure not least because organisations that are subject to constant change and upheaval find it hard to be efficient and effective. We considered these changes in detail in the previous chapter. Here we are concerned with their effect on the work of health professionals.

McDONALDISATION

The sociologist, George Ritzer, summed up the changes wrought on service industries by managerialism by describing them as '**McDonaldisation**' (2011). Ritzer says that to understand McDonaldisation we first have to understand the sociologist Max Weber's work on **rationality**, particularly, his analysis of the benefits and drawbacks of the rise of bureaucracy. Weber described **bureaucracies** as highly formalised, impersonal organisations which based all decision-making on what Weber called 'calculative' rationality. 'Calculative' rationality involved impersonal cost–benefit analysis based on economic calculations. Weber saw this form of 'calculative' rationality as supplanting earlier forms of rationality based in culture, tradition, human values and relationships. He also saw this type of rationality as an 'iron cage' which reduced each worker to a 'cog' in an impersonal bureaucratic machine (Weber, 2019). Ritzer (2011) believed that the social process that he called McDonaldisation involved an attempt to more fully subjugate human service occupations to the calculative rationality described by Weber. What he calls 'McDonaldism' has four dimensions which mirror the dimensions of bureaucratic rationality described by Weber.

- **Efficiency** – cutting costs: speeding up work, shifting service costs onto customers
- **Calculability** – quantification: cost benefit analysis, audits, performance measurement
- **Predictability** – standardisation of work, products and services
- **Increased control** – achieved by replacing or controlling humans with non-human technologies such as robots, digital technologies, artificial intelligence (AI)

Ritzer says that McDonalds wanted to introduce a conveyer belt system into its outlets to increase its profits. To facilitate this, they introduced standardised products to eliminate individual choice by consumers. They also standardised and speeded up customer service by scripting interactions with customers, such as 'do you want fries with that' or 'have a nice day'. Finally, they saw another opportunity to reduce staff and increase profits by 'putting customers to work' filling their own cups with drinks and clearing their own tables. We see McDonaldisation in healthcare in the standardisation of care delivery; the increased burden of audit; the relentless focus on throughput and the pressure on patients to 'self-manage' their illnesses (Dorsey & Ritzer, 2016).

Ritzer suggests that McDonaldisation has irrational consequences. For example, it has inbuilt inefficiencies, such as increasing waste and litter through the use of disposable products. These costs to the planet are not picked up by McDonalds but by the public (Ritzer, 2011). Similarly, in healthcare, managerialist reforms have led to many items of equipment, such as personal protective equipment (PPE), once produced locally or in house, being outsourced to the global market. This has both affected the security of supply (as became obvious during the COVID-19 pandemic) and led to an exponential increase in the use of single use, disposable products with serious implications for the environment (Hasan & Harley, 2021). Dorsey and Ritzer (2016) suggest that other inefficiencies in healthcare include dehumanising patients, demoralising frontline staff and increasing burnout, affecting both the effectiveness of care and staff turnover. In the next section, we turn to look at the changing nature of nursing work and we will think about how managerialism has affected what nurses do.

REFLECTION POINT

We have discussed Ritzer's concept of McDonaldisation. Can you think of examples of McDonaldisation from your own experiences of healthcare? Are there any advantages to McDonaldising healthcare? Can you think of examples of the 'inbuilt inefficiencies' identified by Ritzer?

The Changing Nature of Nursing Work

THE ORIGINS OF NURSING

Nursing developed as a professional occupation at the end of the nineteenth century, achieving state registration in 1919 as we saw earlier. There were various reasons for the development of the nursing profession, amongst which was the growth of the hospital system during the nineteenth century. This led to the call from doctors for a well-trained new assistant due to the growing volume and complexity of medical work (Dingwall et al., 2002). In addition, Victorian society was increasingly concerned about the moral and physical health of the poor in industrial cities, so social reformers were keen to develop an occupation that would bring instruction about hygiene to the poor (Dean & Bolton, 1980). There was also a moral panic about 'surplus women' after the 1851 census revealed an excess of women in the population and suggested that almost half a million 'surplus' women would be unable to marry. Concerns centred not only on how they would support themselves but also on how they would be managed without a husband to control them (Worsnop, 1990). As the campaign for women's suffrage developed in the latter half of the nineteenth century there was also increasing pressure from women campaigners to develop occupations that would allow women to support themselves independently (Hawkins, 2010).

Into these debates came nursing reformers, such as Florence Nightingale. She proposed the creation of a 'new model nurse' based on a gendered division of labour in which doctors and nurses would occupy 'separate spheres' just as men and women did in the home. Nursing's vocation would be to care both for the patient and his environment; methodically observing patients; carrying out treatments ordered by doctors and acting with 'intelligent obedience' (Nightingale, 1860). Nurses would also exemplify and promote high moral standards (Nightingale, 1990). Nightingale and her fellow reformers' conception of the 'new model nurse' was a compromise between progressive and conservative forces in Victorian society. Thus, nursing would provide an assistant to doctors; a means to cleanse and morally instruct the poor and respectable employment for the 'surplus' woman. While this would give these women careers, they would nevertheless be institutionally contained and controlled within nurses' homes. Strict discipline was central to early nurse reformers' conception of nursing. Nightingale, like other nurse reformers from her class, saw themselves as commanding this new nursing workforce, just as married ladies from their class commanded their domestic servants (Brooks, 2001).

Nursing as women's Work

We can see therefore that the original nursing reformers had a strongly gendered conception of nursing. According to Florence Nightingale, in a letter to trainee nurses at St Thomas' Hospital; 'to be a good nurse one must be a good woman'. She then advised them to exhibit virtues of quietness, gentleness, patience, endurance, forbearance, obedience and thoroughness, striving to be 'good' rather than 'clever' nurses (Nightingale, 1990). We see here that nurses were expected by Nightingale to display traits, such as empathy, subordination and compliance, consistent with the gender order described by Connell (2009) (see Chapter 3). Being a good nurse was conceptualised as a matter of feminine character more than skill, intelligence or education.

An early feminist analysis of nursing by Gamarnikow (1991) argued that early nursing reformers believed that the division of labour between nurses and doctors should be based on 'natural' differences between men and women. This was consistent with their aspiration for nursing to occupy a separate feminine sphere. Gamarnikow (1991) suggested that the roles of doctor, nurse and patient replicated that of the father, mother and child in the Victorian household. The doctor gave the orders and the nurse would obediently follow instructions seeing that the patient also complied. Patients were expected to accept this unquestioningly and do as they were told. There was no room for either patient involvement or nursing judgement in this patriarchal view of medical practice.

By the late twentieth century, the gender division of healthcare labour was changing and this has continued into the twenty-first century. In 2023, women made up 49% of the medical workforce (GMC, 2023), so Gamarnikow's domestic analogy has become dated. However, men still only make up 10.9% of the nursing workforce. Men have traditionally achieved senior posts more quickly; a phenomenon that has been described as the 'glass escalator'. In 2020, women still filled less than one-third of senior nursing posts and earned 17% less than men in similar roles (Clayton-Hathaway et al., 2020).

The rise of 'second-wave' feminism' in the 1960s and 1970s had some influence on nursing policy and politics. Feminist writers in this era debated whether the route to advancement for nursing lay in taking over tasks from doctors or whether it lay in promoting a new understanding of the importance of what nurses do; namely, caring. The feminist sociologist, Ann Oakley, argued that nurses needed to assert the importance of the caring work that they did as well as the skill it involved (Oakley, 1984). This was part of a much bigger debate not only about the failure of society to properly value women's work but also about society's denigration of more feminine, person-centred values. These issues have now become part of a wider debate about the need to protect the values of altruism and compassion (which had informed the creation of the NHS) from neoliberalism and managerialism's focus on cost-cutting and efficiency (Ballatt et al., 2020). The question for nurses was; could nursing teach society to properly understand and value caring or would the status of nursing only rise if nurses chose more masculine career aspirations? This latter option would involve embracing either a more managerial role or a technical role as a doctor substitute, whilst handing over bedside care to a lower-paid grade of worker.

From the 1960s onwards there were moves to professionalise nursing. Nursing leaders in this era took a credentialist approach to raising nursing's professional status. In 1972, the 'Briggs Report' made a number of recommendations to modernise and professionalise nursing. It advocated a single unitary nursing regulator. This resulted in the creation of the United Kingdom Central Council (UKCC) which existed from 1983 until it was replaced by the NMC in 2002. Briggs also recommended that nursing became a research-based profession with better education for nurses and a higher proportion of degree-educated nurses (Dingwall et al., 2002). This report started the reform of nurse education that eventually led to it becoming an all-graduate profession in 2013.

A great deal of nursing scholarship has tried to analyse what it is that nurses do in an attempt to both define nursing and demonstrate its value. One of the discourses within this literature asserts the continued importance of person-centred care and of nurses' emotion work with patients; this discourse has strong links with the sociology of care. This discourse not only asserts the importance of bedside care; it also stresses the skill and complexity involved in that care (Smith, 2011). Another discourse promotes the technical aspects of nursing and suggests that its connection with caring is outdated; nursing is no longer a 'practical' occupation or a 'vocation'. It is instead a 'highly technically skilled' and 'evidence-based' occupation allied to medicine (Garcia & Qureshi, 2022). A further discourse emphasises nursing's pivotal place in healthcare organisations, linking nursing to the values of managerialism. It emphasises nursing's managerial work, such as meeting organisational targets and managing patient pathways to increase throughput (Allen, 2018). It is clear, therefore, that nursing roles are many faceted and that numerous debates have centred on the relative importance of different parts of the nursing role, such as bedside care, technical tasks and management, as well as the balance between them. We will look in a little more detail at these different components of nursing work next.

WHAT DO NURSES DO?

There have been many attempts to define nursing. One of the classic definitions of nursing was first given in the 1950s by Virginia Henderson. She said of nursing:

'Nursing is primarily helping people (sick or well) in the performance of those activities contributing to health, or its recovery (or to a peaceful death) that they would perform unaided if they had the necessary strength, will, or knowledge. It is likewise the unique contribution of nursing to help people to be independent of such assistance as soon as possible…'.

(Henderson, 1978, p. 121)

The UK nursing regulator does not define nursing and its conception of what nursing is has to be inferred from its code of conduct and its publication; 'Standards of Proficiency for Registered Nurses' (NMC, 2018). In the latest NMC Code (2018) we see that nurses are still held accountable for the delivery of what it calls the 'fundamentals of care'. However, we have seen progressive change in how the NMC conceives of nursing with both these documents placing a far greater emphasis on nurses' managerial responsibilities than earlier documents.

Nursing authors have tried for many years to grapple with what nurses do and identify the different parts of their work. In a classic paper, James (1992), proposed a **'care formula'** to describe nursing. She said that nursing care consisted of **physical labour, emotional labour and organisation**.

A more recent model of nursing work by Jackson et al. (2021), based on a meta-narrative review, identified the same three components as James. However, they added another component of nursing work which they described as **'cognitive work'**. This recognises that nurses need to employ complex cognitive and critical thinking skills when, for example, assessing patients and prioritising care. Thus, we can see nursing as having four components:

Nursing = Physical work + Emotion work + Cognitive work + Organisational work

These formulae offer a useful way to think about what nurses do. Many of the debates about the role of nurses have focused on the balance between these four components of nursing. Below is an example of the complexity of what nurses do. Then we will look at the components of nursing work in a little more detail.

Case Example: The Complexity of Nursing Work

The organisation theorist, Peter Frost, described a nurse whose care he had watched while he was in hospital being treated for cancer. A patient opposite him had had a gastrectomy and oesophagectomy; was struggling to recover and to cope with his feeding tube and had been incontinent on the way to the bathroom. Frost said he looked 'shaken, humiliated and dejected'. The new nurse on duty had been watching him constantly while attending to other patients. She quickly intervened, assessed him, carried out technical care tasks and organised other professionals to review and treat him. She spent time with him, held his hand, spoke comfortingly, explained the care she was arranging and encouraged him to feel more optimistic. She was physically present at his bedside at regular intervals throughout the shift. Importantly, Frost says, she was willing to step out of her standard routine to address the needs of a patient who she saw was in trouble. By the end of her shift he was looking more cheerful and confident. He confided in Frost that before this nurse had come on duty he had felt that 'his last day had come'.

(Frost, 1999)

Physical Work

The traditional understanding of nursing care associates it with what the NMC calls the 'fundamentals of care'. The NMC Code (2018) describes these as:

'The fundamentals of care include, but are not limited to, nutrition, hydration, bladder and bowel care, physical handling and making sure that those receiving care are kept in clean and hygienic conditions. It includes making sure that those receiving care have adequate access to nutrition and

hydration, and making sure that you provide help to those who are not able to feed themselves or drink fluid unaided'.

These fundamental care tasks have been subsumed by sociologists under the term **'body work'**. This describes work which involves handling of and close contact with people's bodies and with bodily fluids. It is, therefore, work that also involves physical intimacy (Twigg, 2006). Body work has had a problematic status in many cultures, being associated with 'dirty' and low-status work; particularly when this work involves dealing with leaking bodies. As we saw in Chapter 5, body leakage is perceived as 'matter out of place' and therefore polluting (Douglas, 2003). The sociologist, Everett Hughes, said that certain types of jobs could be viewed as **'dirty' work** that carried stigma and evoked social disgust. 'Dirty' jobs were jobs that were essential to society but that society would sooner not think about (Hughes, 1962). 'Dirtiness' is a social construction and work is labelled 'dirty' because it is perceived as violating certain cultural norms thus carrying physical, social or moral 'taint' (Ashforth & Kreiner, 1999). Ashforth and Kreiner suggest that occupations engaging in 'dirty' work require strong occupational cultures that assert the importance and dignity of what they do.

Writers on body work in nursing have emphasised the importance and complexity of what nurses do when they carry out body work and its privileged nature (Wolf, 2014). Much of this work draws on sociological ideas, particularly interactionism and phenomenology. Lawler has argued that our bodies are not just objects but our means of expression and identity. Trouble in our bodies can be threatening to our sense of personhood. Nurses do not just care for the objective body; they also negotiate a delicate social terrain to maintain the patient's privacy, dignity and sense of personhood (Draper, 2014). This involves both explicit and tacit knowledge and these are complex skills that need to be learned (Kontos & Naglie, 2009). Nurses, according to Lawler, have designed a range of strategies to create protective and private spaces to minimise the patient's shame and embarrassment and protect their sense of self (Lawler, 2006). Thus, maintaining the patient's sense of self requires person-centred rather than task-centred care (Wolf, 2014). Similarly, Twigg (2006), has suggested that it is part of the symbolic work of nursing to mediate the pollution of dealing with sick bodies by transforming the meaning of bodily care from 'dirty' tasks to personal acts of caring.

Despite these arguments for the importance and skill of body work there has been a steady move away from body work by registered nurses towards either management tasks or more technical tasks delegated by doctors. A number of authors have also identified a trend for occupations to move away from 'dirty' work in a bid to enhance their status; by, for example, delegating body work to lower grades, in favour of cleaner, 'hands off' tasks (Bjørk, 1995). However, this move away from body work may not be chosen by nurses. Wolf (2014) suggests that as health systems increase their demands on nurses there is increasing pressure on them to move away from the bedside. Wolf says this is a 'seductive' pressure on nurses, some of whom will see an opportunity to raise their status by becoming 'information managers'. On the other hand, Lundin Gurné et al. (2021) describe registered nurses in Sweden as striving against these demands in order to maintain their closeness to patients.

Daykin and Clarke (2000) have argued that these changes have largely been due to managerial changes in work organisation; including changing shift patterns and skill mix in an attempt to get 'more for less' from the nursing workforce. Registered nurses have been substituted with cheaper grades of worker, such as healthcare assistants. Daykin and Clarke observe that these changes involve the deskilling and routinisation of work; work becomes task focused rather than patient focused and the pace and intensity of work is increased. Fundamental care largely becomes the domain of the healthcare assistant and registered nurses may have little time to supervise it. Sociologists of work describe these changes as 'work intensification' (Cooke, 2006a) and they are the result of Taylorist controls on nursing work (Wong, 2004).

Kitson et al. (2014) suggest that nurses and healthcare assistants are forced into a 'task and time' mentality in which getting through the work is more important than engaging with the patient. As a result, care becomes depersonalised, and the patient's body is objectified; this can lead to the patient feeling 'ignored, humiliated and unsafe' (Kitson, 2018). Kitson also suggests that nurses' dissatisfaction with their inability to deliver good-quality care is a major cause of nursing burnout.

Emotion Work

The term 'emotional labour' was first used by the sociologist Arlie Hochschild to describe the work of flight attendants (Hochschild, 2012). She defines emotional labour as:

> *'The induction or suppression of feeling in order to sustain an outward appearance that produces in others a sense of being cared for' (p. 7).*

Hochschild's key point about emotion work is that in service industries it is seen as a valuable commercial asset and so has been brought under the control of managers. In the airline industry, managers started to closely manage workers' emotional labour, enforcing an expectation of 'genuinely friendly' service whilst instructing flight attendants to always 'think sales'. The contradiction between the instruction to be 'genuine' and to 'think sales' and the pressure to present a corporate demeanour could make flight attendants feel fake and insincere. Hochschild described how the creation of budget airlines and 'industry speed up' then led flight attendants to start to feel increased pressure and alienation. This alienation resulted from being expected to continue to maintain a warm and friendly demeanour while their work intensified; the service they could deliver deteriorated and passengers became more dissatisfied and aggressive. They began to feel that their emotions and how they expressed them were no longer under their control and some coped with the stress by going into 'robot' mode.

Smith (2011) has developed Hochschild's ideas in relation to nursing, but she argues that emotional labour in nursing has a different status to that of the flight attendants studied by Hochschild. She asserts that nursing is a profession so nurses' emotional labour has been given freely by nurses as an expression of their professional values. She also argues that emotion work is hard work but that it is often invisible and undervalued. This is because it is seen as 'natural' women's work and thus seen as an expression of 'womanly' character requiring no skill or knowledge. Smith refutes this assumption and her book examines the complex and challenging emotional situations that nurses have to deal with; handling not only anxiety, pain, grief, frustration and death but also anger and aggression from patients and relatives.

Like Kitson (2018) Smith argues that emotion work is inseparable from the delivery of fundamental care. Emotion work is, in part, about building a relationship with a patient; treating them with respect; listening to their concerns and offering encouragement, reassurance and information. However, for Smith, actions are even more important than words. It is in attentiveness to the 'little things' that nurses express such care. For example, making sure a patient's hair and nails are cared for; hearing aid working and spectacles clean (Smith, 2012).

Like body work, emotion work can be under threat from the pressure on nurses to move away from the bedside as well as the 'industry speed up' described by Hochschild (2012). This is experienced by nurses as the 'task and time' pressures described by Kitson (2014). The 'gestures of care' described by Smith (2012) can get lost when care is speeded up and routinised as we saw above when talking about bodily care. Then, care staff can go into 'robot' mode like Hochschild's flight attendants. Communications can also become superficial when care is routinised and then we may see the superficial scripted interactions familiar to us from McDonaldised settings; the nursing equivalents of, 'do you want fries with that'.

Cognitive Work

Jackson et al. (2021) identified nurses' cognitive work as requiring lifelong **acquisition of knowledge** as nurses adapt to new demands. Nurses learn both through experience and through study. Nurses progress from novice to expert practitioner as they continue to develop their theoretical and experiential knowledge (Benner, 2001). Jackson et al. (2021) also suggest that nurses' cognitive work involves **critical thinking skills**, in particular, clinical reasoning, problem solving and clinical decision-making. Jackson and others also identify cognitive work linked to nurses' organisational duties; nurses typically need to manage a large number of competing demands and interruptions creating a high cognitive load. **Managing a high cognitive load** requires an ability to stack tasks; continually assess and reassess their urgency and reprioritise them as circumstances evolve. They describe these various types of cognitive work as a substantial part of nurses' overall work requiring both education and intelligence.

For example, we saw above that attentiveness to the patient's needs is important to ensure patient's physical needs are met and that they feel safe and cared for. **Vigilance** and attentiveness to a patient's condition can also be vital to patient safety. Vigilance involves being watchful for possible danger to the patient. Meyer and Lavin (2005) point out that this also means being able to properly interpret the meaning and significance of cues, such as changes in a patient's vital signs, appearance or behaviour. This involves understanding which cues are clinically significant; being able to assess the risks in practice situations, and making appropriate clinical decisions in response to risks. Importantly, this also involves being able to piece cues together in a process described as **'pattern recognition'** (Benner, 2001). Interpreting the meaning of cues involves both knowledge and experience and thus is more highly developed in the expert nurse. Being able to make sound clinical decisions also requires having time to think; this can be negatively affected by routinising and speeding up care.

A considerable number of studies have indicated that patient outcomes (in particular, mortality rates) are better in settings where there are more registered nurses (Aiken et al., 2014) and also where nurses are more highly educated (Aiken et al., 2011). A higher level of registered nurse staffing has been shown to reduce the incidence of staff failing to pick up cues, leading to a **'failure to rescue'** patients from preventable deterioration or death from conditions such as pneumonia, shock, gastrointestinal bleeding and sepsis. This demonstrates the importance of nurses' cognitive work; particularly as expressed in nursing vigilance (Shever, 2011). However, where registered nurses are dealing with competing organisational demands, which take them away from the patient bedside, then the opportunities to exercise nursing vigilance are reduced. As discussed earlier, studies have suggested that this cognitive work by nurses cannot be fully replaced by standardised approaches, such as the early warning score, delivered by lower grades of worker (Odell et al., 2009).

Organisational Work

A number of studies have highlighted nurses' organisational work, in particular their role in coordinating patient care. This role has become more central as patient care has become more complex and fast paced. Latimer's (2000) ethnographic study of medical wards described nurses as the 'conductors' of care who managed patients' pathways through the institution (see Chapter 10). Allen (2014) has argued that nurses need to recognise that organisation is now a central part of the nurse's role and cease hoping for a world where nurses can deliver 'holistic care' as articulated by authors such as Smith (2012).

Allen (2018) argues that nurses are the 'glue' in healthcare systems who coordinate the patient's treatment. Nurses achieve this not only through aligning and integrating activities, such as tests and treatments, but also through what Allen calls **'translation'**; Allen has borrowed this term from **'actor network theory'**. This is a social theory originating in technology. It is a social constructionist theory which sees society as accomplished through individuals acting in networks. The concept of 'translation' refers to the ways in which individual actors interpret and define problems in ways that mobilise the activities of others. Allen uses the example of the ways in which ward nurses clarify the responsibilities of junior doctors. Thus, Allen sees nurses' central role as **'the mobilisation of health trajectories'**, that is, coordinating and accomplishing the patient's pathway through the institution through information management.

Jackson et al. (2021) noted that nurses spent around half of their time either in consultation with other professionals or documenting care. They suggest that Allen has done a service to nurses in highlighting the importance of their organisational work rather than treating it as a distraction from the 'real' work of nursing. However, Allen's model of nurses' organisational work leaves little room for nurses' organisation and supervision of bedside care. In producing her care formula, James (1992) had described organisation as being about ensuring that the balance of physical and emotional labour was maintained and that the details of care were attended to. She said that it was in 'the minutiae of daily life' that nurses' organisation skills maintained the quality of care. Nurses have similarly described maintaining high quality of care as being about attentiveness to the 'little things' (Cooke, 2006b). James (1992) concludes by discussing both the importance and difficulty of balancing the different components of care. This is a dilemma that nursing has always faced but perhaps does so most acutely in an era of managerialism and austerity.

The historian Susan Reverby said the dilemma for nursing is that it has been 'ordered to care' by a society that refuses to value caring (Reverby, 1987). Despite this, many nurses have continued to assert the value of caring (Watson, 2019). According to Davies (1995), nursing's professional 'predicament' is that much of what nurses do is unrecognised. She suggests that healthcare has a masculine view of professionalism and that most of the caring work that nurses do is unacknowledged. Doctors, politicians and managers simply fail to see it. Instead, it is the visible things that nurses do, such as producing documentation and managing bed flow, that are audited and rewarded. Nurses are increasingly seen by managers and politicians as too expensive to be 'wasted' on bedside care. This has led to nurses being pulled away from the bedside by other demands, yet they are still being held accountable for the fundamentals of care. Increasingly, bedside care has been seen by managers and policymakers as low-skill work that can be delegated to low-waged staff and yet nurses remain accountable for that care. When care fails, it is often nurses that are blamed. In our final chapter, we will consider situations where care fails.

REFLECTION POINT

Nursing = Physical work + Emotion work + Cognitive work + Organisational work

Look back at the case example at the start of this section and identify the different components of nursing work that it demonstrates. Thinking about your own experience of nursing work, do you think that the formula above fully describes nursing work? If not, how would you change it? How would you assess the relative importance of these four components of nursing work? Are there any components of nursing work that you think are neglected? Why?

Summary of Key Points

- Traditional ideas of professionalism have been increasingly challenged. Most professionals now work in institutions where they are subject to close managerial and bureaucratic controls.
- Managerialism is now a dominant feature of public services. Managerialism can be characterised by increased focus on standardisation, predictability, cost efficiency and managerial control. This has also been described as 'McDonaldisation'.

- Nursing involves 'body work', emotional labour, cognitive work and organisational work.
- There have been debates about the boundaries of nursing and the relative importance of different components of the nurse's role. The boundaries of nursing have often been decided by other powerful groups such as doctors, managers and politicians.

Further Reading

Ballatt, J., Campling, P., & Maloney, C. (2020). *Intelligent kindness: Rehabilitating the welfare state*. Cambridge University Press.
Dorsey, E. R., & Ritzer, G. (2016). The McDonaldization of medicine. *JAMA Neurology, 73*(1), 15–16.
Smith, P. (2011). *The emotional labour of nursing revisited: Can nurses still care?* Bloomsbury Publishing.
Watson, C. (2019). *The language of kindness: A nurse's story*. Penguin Books.

References

Abbasi, K. (2023). Junior doctors' anger can no longer be ignored. *BMJ, 380*, 425.
Aiken, L. H., Cimiotti, J. P., Sloane, D. M., Smith, H. L., Flynn, L., & Neff, D. F. (2011). The effects of nurse staffing and nurse education on patient deaths in hospitals with different nurse work environments. *Medical Care, 49*(12), 1047.
Aiken, L. H., Sloane, D. M., Bruyneel, L., Van den Heede, K., Griffiths, P., Busse, R., & Sermeus, W. (2014). Nurse staffing and education and hospital mortality in nine European countries: A retrospective observational study. *The Lancet, 383*(9931), 1824–1830.
Allen, D. (2014). *The invisible work of nurses: Hospitals, organisation and healthcare*. Routledge.
Allen, D. (2018). Translational mobilisation theory: A new paradigm for understanding the organisational elements of nursing work. *International Journal of Nursing Studies, 79*, 36–42.
Ashforth, B. E., & Kreiner, G. E. (1999). "How can you do it?": Dirty work and the challenge of constructing a positive identity. *Academy of Management Review, 24*(3), 413–434.
Aufhauser, R. K. (1973). Slavery and scientific management. *The Journal of Economic History, 33*(4), 811–824.
Ballatt, J., Campling, P., & Maloney, C. (2020). *Intelligent kindness: Rehabilitating the welfare state*. Cambridge University Press.
Benner, P. E. (2001). *From novice to expert: Excellence and power in clinical nursing practice*. Pearson.
Bjørk, I. T. (1995). Neglected conflicts in the discipline of nursing: Perceptions of the importance and value of practical skill. *Journal of Advanced Nursing, 22*(1), 6–12.
Braddock, R., Mahony, P., & Taylor, P. A. (2006). Globalisation, commercialisation, managerialism and internationalisation: Challenges for higher education in the developing world. *The International Journal of Learning, 13*(8), 61–67.
Brooks, J. (2001). Structured by class, bound by gender. *International History of Nursing Journal, 6*(2), 13.
Cheraghi-Sohi, S., & Calnan, M. (2013). Discretion or discretions? Delineating professional discretion: The case of English medical practice. *Social Science & Medicine, 96*, 52–59.
Clayton-Hathway, K., Humbert, A. L., Schut, S., McIlroy, R., & Griffiths, H. (2020). *Gender and Nursing as a profession: Valuing nurses and paying them their worth*. Royal College of Nursing.
Connell, R. (2009). *Gender*. Polity Press.
Cooke, B. (2003). The denial of slavery in management studies. *Journal of Management Studies, 40*(8), 1895–1918.
Cooke, H. (2006a). Seagull management and the control of nursing work. *Work, Employment and Society, 20*(2), 223–243.
Cooke, H. (2006b). The surveillance of nursing standards: An organisational case study. *International Journal of Nursing Studies, 43*(8), 975–984.
Crompton, R. (1990). Professions in the current context. *Work, Employment and Society, 4*(5), 147–166.
Davies, C. (1995). *Gender and the professional predicament in nursing*. McGraw-Hill Education.
Daykin, N., & Clarke, B. (2000). 'They'll still get the bodily care'. Discourses of care and relationships between nurses and health care assistants in the NHS. *Sociology of Health & Illness, 22*(3), 349–363.
Dean, M., & Bolton, G. (1980). The administration of poverty and the development of nursing practice in nineteenth-century England. In Davies, C. (Ed.), *Rewriting Nursing History* (pp. 76–101). Croom Helm Ltd.

Dingwall, R., Rafferty, A. M., & Webster, C. (2002). *An introduction to the social history of nursing.* Routledge.

Dorsey, E. R., & Ritzer, G. (2016). The McDonaldization of medicine. *JAMA Neurology, 73*(1), 15–16.

Douglas, M. (2003). *Purity and danger: An analysis of concepts of pollution and taboo.* Routledge.

Draper, J. (2014). Embodied practice: Rediscovering the 'heart' of nursing. *Journal of Advanced Nursing, 70*(10), 2235–2244.

Durkheim, E. (2013). *Professional ethics and civic morals.* Routledge.

Evetts, J. (2011). A new professionalism? Challenges and opportunities. *Current Sociology, 59*(4), 406–422.

Flexner, A. (2001). Is social work a profession? *Research on Social Work Practice, 11*(2), 152–165.

Fothergill, L. J., Al-Oraibi, A., Houdmont, J., Conway, J., Evans, C., Timmons, S., & Blake, H. (2022). Nation-wide evaluation of the advanced clinical practitioner role in England: A cross-sectional survey. *BMJ Open, 12*(1), e055475.

Freidson, E. (1983). The reorganization of the professions by regulation. *Law and Human Behavior, 7*(2–3), 279–290.

Freidson, E. (1988). *Profession of medicine: A study of the sociology of applied knowledge.* University of Chicago Press.

Freidson, E. (2001). *Professionalism, the third logic: On the practice of knowledge.* University of Chicago Press.

Freund, P., McGuire, M., & Podhurst, L. (2003). *Health, illness and the social body: A critical sociology* (4th ed.). Prentice-Hall.

Frost, P. J. (1999). Why compassion counts!. *Journal of Management Inquiry, 8*(2), 127–133.

Gamarnikow, E. (1991). Nurse or woman: Gender and professionalism in reformed nursing 1860–1923. In Holden, P., & Littlewood, J. (Eds.), *Anthropology and Nursing* (pp. 110–129). Routledge.

Garcia, R., & Qureshi, I. (2022). Nurse identity: Reality and media portrayal. *Evidence-Based Nursing, 25*(1), 1–5.

Germov, J. (2005). Managerialism in the Australian public health sector: Towards the hyper-rationalisation of professional bureaucracies. *Sociology of Health & Illness, 27*(6), 738–758.

Gerth, H. H., & Mills, C. W. (Eds.). (2014). *From max weber: Essays in sociology.* Routledge.

GMC. (2023). *The state of medical education and practice in the UK: The workforce report.* Retrieved January 22, 2024, from https://www.gmc-uk.org/-/media/documents/workforce-report-2023-full-report_pdf-103569478.pdf.

Greenwood, E. (1957). Attributes of a profession. *Social Work, 2*(3), 45–55.

Hafferty, F. W., & Castellani, B. (2010). The increasing complexities of professionalism. *Academic Medicine, 85*(2), 288–301.

Hallett, C., & Cooke, H. (2011). *Historical investigations into the professional self-regulation of nursing: Vol. 1 Nursing.* Nursing and Midwifery Council.

Hasan, A., & Harley, K. (2021). Solution not pollution! How can we make the NHS more sustainable? *Faculty Dental Journal, 12*(2), 82–85.

Hawkins, S. (2010). *Nursing and women's labour in the nineteenth century: The quest for independence.* Routledge.

Henderson, V. (1978). The concept of nursing. *Journal of Advanced Nursing, 3*(2), 113–130.

Hochschild, A. R. (2012). *The managed heart* (3rd ed.). University of California Press.

Hood, C. (1991). A public management for all seasons? *Public Administration, 69*, 3–19.

Hooks, C., & Walker, S. (2020). An exploration of the role of advanced clinical practitioners in the East of England. *British Journal of Nursing, 29*(15), 864–869.

Hughes, E. C. (1962). Good people and dirty work. *Social Problems, 10*(1), 3–11.

Hughes, J. C., Bamford, C., & May, C. (2008). Types of centredness in health care: themes and concepts. *Medicine, Health Care and Philosophy, 11*, 455–463.

Jackson, J., Anderson, J., & Maben, J. (2021). What is nursing work? A meta-narrative review and integrated framework. *International Journal of Nursing Studies, 122*, 103944.

James, N. (1992). Care= organisation+ physical labour+ emotional labour. *Sociology of Health & Illness, 14*(4), 488–509.

Jamous, H., & Peloille, B. (1970). Changes in the French university-hospital system. In Jackson, J. (Ed.), *Professions and professionalization* (pp. 111–152). Cambridge University Press.

Johnson, T. J. (2016). *Professions and power.* Routledge.

Kitson, A. L. (2018). The fundamentals of care framework as a point-of-care nursing theory. *Nursing Research, 67*(2), 99–107.

Kitson, A., Muntlin Athlin, A., & Conroy, T. (2014). Anything but basic: Nursing's challenge in meeting patients' fundamental care needs. *Journal of Nursing Scholarship, 46*(5), 331–339.

Klikauer, T. (2015). What is managerialism? *Critical Sociology, 41*(7–8), 1103–1119.

Kontos P.C. & Naglie G. (2009). Tacit knowledge of caring and embodied selfhood. *Sociology of Health & Illness, 31*(5), 688–704.

Larson, M. (2012). *The rise of professionalism: Monopolies of competence and sheltered markets*. Transaction Publishers.

Latimer, J. E. (2000). *The conduct of care: Understanding nursing practice*. John Wiley & Sons.

Lawler, J. (2006). *Behind the screens: Nursing, somology, and the problem of the body*. Sydney University Press.

Lawrence, C. (2006). *Medicine in the making of modern Britain, 1700–1920*. Routledge.

Lightfoot, L. (2016). *The student experience–then and now*. The Guardian. 24th June. Retrieved August 08, 2023, from https://www.theguardian.com/education/2016/jun/24/has-university-life-changed-student-experience-past-present-parents-vox-pops#:~:text=.

Lundin Gurné, F., Lidén, E., Jakobsson Ung, E., Kirkevold, M., Öhlén, J., & Jakobsson, S (2021). Striving to be in close proximity to the patient: An interpretive descriptive study of nursing practice from the perspectives of clinically experienced registered nurses. *Nursing Inquiry, 28*(2), e12387.

McCartney, M. (2011). Well enough to work? *BMJ, 342*, d599.

McKinlay, J. B., & Marceau, L. D. (2002). The end of the golden age of doctoring. *International Journal of Health Services, 32*(2), 379–416.

McKinlay, J. B., & Stoeckle, J. D. (2020). Corporatization and the social transformation of doctoring. *The Corporate Transformation of Health Care, 133–149.*

Meyer, G., & Lavin, M. A. (2005). Vigilance: The essence of nursing. *Online Journal of Issues in Nursing, 10*(3), 8.

NHS England. (2017). *Multi-professional framework for advanced clinical practice in England*. Health Education England. https://www.hee.nhs.uk/sites/default/files/documents/multi-professionalframeworkforad-vancedclinicalpracticeinengland.pdf.

Nightingale, F. (1860). *Notes on nursing: What it is, and what it is not*. D. Appleton and Company. Retrieved January 22, 2024, from https://digital.library.upenn.edu/women/nightingale/nursing/nursing.html.

Nightingale, F. (1990). *Ever yours, Florence Nightingale: Selected letters*. Harvard University Press.

NMC. (2018). *Future nurse: Standards of proficiency for registered nurses*. Retrieved January 22, 2024, from https://www.nmc.org.uk/globalassets/sitedocuments/nmc-publications/nmc-code.pdf.

Noordegraaf, M. (2007). From "pure" to "hybrid" professionalism: Present-day professionalism in ambiguous public domains. *Administration & Society, 39*(6), 761–785. https://www.nmc.org.uk/globalassets/sitedocu-ments/nmc-publications/nmc-code.pdf.

Nursing & Midwifery Council (NMC). (2018). *The code: Professional standards of practice and behaviour for nurses, midwives and nursing associates*. Retrieved January 22, 2024, from http://www.nmc.org.uk/globalas-sets/sitedocuments/nmc-publications/revised-new-nmc-code.pdf.

Oakley, A. (1984). What price professionalism? The importance of being a nurse. *Nursing Times, 80*(50), 24–27.

Odell, M., Victor, C., & Oliver, D. (2009). Nurses' role in detecting deterioration in ward patients: Systematic literature review. *Journal of Advanced Nursing, 65*(10), 1992–2006.

Osborne, D., & Gaebler, T. (1993). *Reinventing government*. Penguin Books.

Piketty, T. (2014). *Capital in the twenty-first century*. Harvard University Press.

Polanyi, M. (1958). *Personal knowledge: "Towards a post-critical philosophy"*. University of Chicago Press.

Porter, S. (1998). *Social theory and nursing practice*. Bloomsbury Publishing.

Reverby, S. (1987). *Ordered to care: The dilemma of American nursing, 1850–1945*. Cambridge University Press.

Ritzer, G. (2011). *The McDonaldization of society*. Pine Forge Press.

Saarni, S., & Gylling, H. (2004). Evidence based medicine guidelines: A solution to rationing or politics disguised as science? *Journal of Medical Ethics, 30*(2), 171.

Shever, L. (2011). The impact of nursing surveillance on failure to rescue. *Research and Theory for Nursing Practice, 25*(2), 107–126.

Simonet, D. (2015). The new public management theory in the British health care system: A critical review. *Administration & Society, 47*(7), 802–826.

Smith, D. C. (1996). The Hippocratic Oath and modern medicine. *Journal of the History of Medicine and Allied Sciences, 51*(4), 484–500.

Smith, P. (2012). *The emotional labour of nursing revisited: Can nurses still care?* Bloomsbury Publishing.

Sotirin, P., Buzzanell, P. M., & Turner, L. H. (2007). Colonizing family: A feminist critique of family management texts. *Journal of Family Communication, 7*(4), 245–263.

Steger, M. B., & Roy, R. K. (2010). *Neoliberalism: A very short introduction.* Oxford University Press.

Taylor, F. W. (2004). *Scientific management.* Routledge.

Twigg, J. (2006). *The body in health and social care.* Bloomsbury Publishing.

UK Government. (2011). *The nursing and midwifery order 2001.* Retrieved January 21, 2024, from https://www.legislation.gov.uk/uksi/2002/253/contents/made.

Watson, C. (2019). *The language of kindness: A nurse's story.* Penguin Random House.

Watson, T. (2017). *Sociology, work and organisation.* Taylor & Francis.

Weber, M. (2019). *Economy and society: A new translation.* Harvard University Press.

Wilensky, H. L. (1964). The professionalization of everyone? *American Journal of Sociology, 70*(2), 137–158.

Wolf, K. A. (2014). Critical perspectives on nursing as bodywork. *Advances in Nursing Science, 37*(2), 147–160.

Wong, W. H. (2004). Caring holistically within new managerialism. *Nursing Inquiry, 11*(1), 2–13.

Worsnop, J. (1990). A re-evaluation of 'the problem of surplus women' in 19th-century England: The case of the 1851 census. *Women's Studies International Forum, 13*(1–2), 21–31.

Healthcare Institutions and Places of Care

Introduction

This chapter looks in more detail at the places where people are cared for. The first part of this chapter looks at the development of the hospital and considers both long-stay institutions and the development of the modern acute hospital. The chapter looks, in particular, at how older people are cared for in hospitals. A central focus of this chapter is how a culture of ageism in healthcare shapes where older people are cared for and what services they receive. The second part of this chapter looks at the development of community care in the UK, focusing on care in the home as well as on the development of the care home sector. It also considers care failures in each sector.

The Hospital as an Institution

THE DEVELOPMENT OF HOSPITALS

There have been hospitals in the UK since the Middle Ages. The earliest were founded by religious orders and offered care but little medical treatment. They were seen as an expression of Christian charity, but, in fact, they were almost certainly a copy of the great Islamic hospitals of the era (Alotaibi, 2021). Many of these religious institutions were destroyed during the Reformation, when the monasteries were dissolved and the UK was forcibly converted to Protestantism by Henry VIII. Many of the major UK hospitals we know today were originally founded in the late eighteenth and early nineteenth centuries, when scientific medicine as we understand it today began to develop. Porter (2004) argues that, at this time, the hospital became the site where new approaches to medicine based on anatomy and physical examination developed.

Nineteenth century hospitals had a large and captive population of 'charity cases' which doctors could use to conduct teaching and research and to refine the practice of their craft. These were the foundations of the private 'voluntary hospitals' that developed in Britain throughout the nineteenth century.

The new hospitals enabled the development of a new **'clinical gaze'** (Foucault, 2002) which, informed by anatomical dissection, looked below the surface of the body and thus divorced the body from the person. According to Foucault, this new 'gaze' was also a new source of power which had both positive and negative consequences. It opened up new possibilities of treatment while at the same time depersonalising patients and cementing doctors' authority over them; we have discussed some of the implications of these changes in Chapters 5, 6 and 9. It was also a masculine gaze which viewed females' bodies as inferior specimens of the male body as we saw in Chapter 4.

In addition to the development of the acute hospital, a range of specialist institutions developed during the nineteenth century to incarcerate 'problem' populations. This coincided with the industrial revolution which required new forms of discipline. We looked at Foucault's (2019) analysis of the disciplinary practices in these institutions in Chapter 5. One example was the new workhouse system. The 1834 Poor Law Amendment Act ended the system of 'parish relief' which had supported the rural poor for centuries and ordered that the poor must only receive relief within workhouses which must have harsher conditions than those suffered by the poorest worker. This was called the principle of 'less eligibility' and it instilled a punitive culture into welfare. Prior to this, the poor were seen as unfortunate victims of economic and social circumstances, but the authors of Poor Law reform asserted that those who were unable to support themselves must be to blame for their misfortunes due to immorality or laziness. The destitute were thus 'undeserving' of all but the harshest forms of assistance (Higginbottom, 2016). Although the intention of the Act was that workhouses would be used to incarcerate and discipline the able-bodied unemployed over time, they were filled by the sick, 'crippled', 'lunatic' and 'idiot' (Dingwall et al., 2002).

Thus, throughout the nineteenth century, specialist institutions were developed to house people labelled as unfit for society, with a huge growth in asylums for the mentally ill as well as institutions to incarcerate people with disabilities, particularly learning disabilities. In the nineteenth and early twentieth centuries the law labelled people with mental health problems and learning disabilities as either 'lunatics', 'idiots' or 'imbeciles'. People thus categorised could be locked away against their will and without their family's consent.

The other influential idea informing this era of incarceration was the theory of population control (later known as 'eugenics') promoted by the economist, Thomas Malthus. Eugenics refers to the theory that human reproduction should be controlled and that 'undesirable' human characteristics should be eliminated from the population. Thomas Malthus believed that poor and 'inferior stock' within the population should be discouraged from breeding. The creation of large-scale bureaucratic institutions to incarcerate 'paupers' and those deemed 'unfit' for society was, in part, inspired by eugenic aims (Englander, 2013). Eugenic theory would later inspire the Nazis, but Shermer (2016) suggests that its ideas had already been extensively employed by UK and US authorities to shut away unwanted people.

Thus, throughout the nineteenth century, hospitals developed along a twin track. On the one hand, acute hospitals provided clinical care and acted as sites for medical research and teaching and, on the other hand, long-stay institutions socially excluded and warehoused the long-term sick and disabled. Many historical studies of these long-stay institutions portray prison-like conditions characterised by poor care and frequent abuse (Burtinshaw & Burt, 2017). For example, the term 'asylum ear' was coined in 1867 to describe the frequent occurrence of haematoma of the ear in asylum inmates. Only much later was it acknowledged that it was due to physical abuse (Oxford English Dictionary, 2023).

LONG-STAY INSTITUTIONS IN THE TWENTIETH CENTURY

As we discussed in Chapter 8, when the NHS was founded in 1948 it took over a patchwork of different types of institution. The problem of what to do with its inheritance of long-stay institutions caring for the mentally ill, older people and people with disabilities became an increasingly pressing concern in the post war period. However, according to Gorsky (2013), NHS leaders failed to prioritise long-stay care and care of older people in resource allocation from the start, choosing instead to favour acute medicine and younger populations.

A movement to put an end to these institutions developed, fuelled by repeated scandals about poor care and institutional abuse (Martin, 1985). In 1961, Goffman (see Chapter 7) conducted an ethnographic study of an asylum for the mentally ill in the US. He described such places as **'total institutions'**. Goffman said that a total institution is any social establishment where 'all aspects of life are conducted in the same place and under the same authority' (p. 17) cut off from the rest of society. Thus, it has the following characteristics:

- People are processed in batches and all treated alike and expected to do the same thing.
- The day is tightly scheduled with the schedule determined, from above, by officials.
- The various enforced activities of the institution are purported to be based on a rational plan which fulfils the aims of the institution (Goffman, 2017).

Goffman argued that, in some respects, total institutions are all alike whether they are a boarding school, prison, asylum or care home. According to Goffman, it is not the aims of the institution that determine the life of an inmate. Instead, it is the institution's need to bureaucratically order the lives of inmates that determines the inmate experience. The desire for order, institutional stability and economy trump any of the institution's aims, however idealistic. Goffman was particularly concerned about the ways in which total institutions strip the inmate of their individual identity; a process he called **'mortification of the self'**. For example, inmates may be stripped of their own clothes and possessions on admission; have limited privacy and their contact with the outside world may be restricted. Goffman found that the inmates of the asylum that he studied had learnt ways to cope with institutional life; some accepted it with resignation and became institutionalised; some became withdrawn; some became intransigent and aggressive; a few found ingenious ways to survive and retain a sense of identity 'in the cracks' of institutional life. Thus, the institution caused new harms to those who were forced to inhabit it; yet, ironically, the coping strategies that inmates employed to cope with institutional life were seen as further proof of their unfitness for society (Goffman, 2017).

Goffman's critique of institutions played an influential part in the movement to speed up the closure of large-scale state institutions such as mental hospitals. Scull (2014) has argued that while the nineteenth century was an era of incarceration, the post war period became an era of **'decarceration'** when long-stay state institutions were progressively closed down and their inmates discharged. Incarceration of inconvenient members of society was an attractive economic proposition in the nineteenth century when labour was cheap and inmates could be forced to work to support the institution. However, in the late twentieth century, these crumbling nineteenth century institutions had become an economic burden. They were difficult and expensive to staff and maintain. They were also prime real estate that could be sold off for a profit. Thus, for Scull, it was not altruism but the drive to cut state spending that eventually led to their demise. As a result, Scull was sceptical about the beneficial results of decarceration. He doubted it would lead to a new 'golden age' of more humane care. Instead, he feared that the moral agenda would be overborne by the economic agenda, leading not to better care but to abandonment and neglect. Thus, according to Carney (2008), following decarceration, mental health services failed to obtain sufficient resources to enable dignified community care.

THE MODERN ACUTE HOSPITAL

More than twenty years ago, Armstrong (1998) suggested that the hospital used to be seen as a vital place for both medical treatment and care and recovery, but times had changed and hospitals and hospital beds had been closed in unprecedented numbers in the period since the 1970s. There has, since this time, been a further steep decline in the number of hospital beds. Instead of inpatient care, many more people are now using hospital services on an 'ambulatory' basis, that is, without staying overnight. The hygiene reforms by Florence Nightingale in the nineteenth century had constituted the hospital as a safe space. According to Nightingale, hospitals should offer the patient a high standard of hygiene and comfort so that s/he was given the best conditions in which to heal. Within the hospital, Nightingale said that space should be carefully managed and divided to promote hygiene and safety, for example, through the use of barrier nursing. Rest was also seen as an important part of the recovery process (McDonald, 2012). However, in the late twentieth century, rest came to be perceived as injurious to health and new health professionals were educated in the 'hazards of immobility'. A new discourse represented the hospital as a place of danger with the risks of cross-infection highlighted to justify discharging patients from the hospital as soon as was conceivably possible. This discourse also justified restricting access to inpatient care, particularly for older people.

Armstrong suggests that this changed function of the hospital can be understood through Foucault's theory of **'governmentality'**. By governmentality, Foucault meant the regulation and control of individual conduct (see Chapter 5). Armstrong saw the changes in hospital care as indicating the rise of a new **'clinical gaze'**. The nineteenth century clinical gaze focused on the body rather than the person (Foucault, 2002). According to Armstrong, the twenty-first-century clinical gaze was set to shift again. It would no longer be focused on the individual patient but on controlling populations. This new clinical gaze is often called **'surveillance medicine'** (see Chapter 1). Healthcare systems refocused their attention towards governing the health and health behaviours of populations. Policymakers advocated moving away from giving direct care and towards surveillance at a distance; the virtual ward is a particularly good example of this. Patients became objects of management rather than care with a new focus on the creation of what Foucault called the **'self-governing subject'**. This refers to the individual who has internalised disciplinary messages that they should engage in 'good' behaviours, that is, self-care and self-management (see Chapter 7). People whose social conditions do not allow them to engage in 'good' behaviours could be blamed or disregarded (Peterson, 2012).

Peterson suggested that there were powerful economic interests shaping changes in health discourses. He saw this change as driven not by a change in medical culture but by economics. He said that the global political economy had played an important role in this new view of the hospital. Managerialism and the pressure to contain healthcare spending had driven the changes in the nature of the acute hospital. We discussed the steady decline in the number of NHS hospital beds in Chapter 8 and, as Armstrong suggests, this has not just been due to the closure of long-stay institutions; many acute hospitals have been closed and acute hospital beds have been severely cut in number. There have been particularly sharp declines in recent years in beds in community hospitals which have traditionally provided rehabilitation, respite and palliative care (Selvan, 2012). These declines have led to overcrowding in emergency departments and a growing concern that a lack of bed capacity may be leading to degradation in the quality of care (Silverskog & Henriksson, 2022). For example, high bed occupancy rates, rapid throughput and frequent moves between wards create the conditions for higher rates of cross-infection as was seen during the COVID-19 pandemic (Castagna et al., 2022). Thus, ironically, it is to some extent, the reform and reconfiguration of modern hospitals that have 'reconstructed' hospital spaces as places of danger (Armstrong, 1998).

As we noted in Chapter 9, we have been encouraged to see the twenty-first-century hospital as a 'garage' service in which patients access a technical fix for a malfunctioning body part. As hospital beds are now a scarce resource, patients are expected to exit the hospital as quickly as possible once 'fixed'. The rise of ambulatory care can have many advantages for younger, fitter and more affluent patients. It can be less suitable for the old, the disabled, those living alone or in deprived circumstances. It leaves less room for care and rehabilitation and can reconstitute the patient who has complications or whose recovery is slower than the planned timetable as a 'problem' patient who has failed to follow the appropriate illness trajectory. We will now consider the implications of this for the older patient.

Ageism, 'Bed Blocking' and the Unwanted Acute Hospital Patient

Ageism refers to stigma, stereotyping, prejudice and discrimination towards others on the basis of age (Pepper, 2015). It is normally directed towards older people and Weir (2023) has suggested that it is the last socially acceptable prejudice; the one remaining '-ism' which goes unchallenged. Ageist stereotypes and age biases pervade our culture and institutions not least within the healthcare system, where it is the most commonly reported type of discrimination (Jonson & Taghizadeh Larsson, 2021). Thus, doctors are less likely to diagnose and treat conditions which are treatable in older people, and services for older people are less well-resourced and staffed (Levy & Apriceno, 2019). Examples of ageism within the healthcare system include talking over the heads of older patients and using 'elderspeak'; a simplified form of speech resembling baby talk when speaking to older people (McLaughlin, 2020). An international systematic review of elder abuse found that it was correlated with social acceptance of age discrimination (WHO, 2022). Thus, age discrimination within healthcare institutions should be a cause for concern.

The 'problem' of 'bed blocking' (or 'delayed discharge') looms large in media discussions of the NHS. It is described as a 'crisis' that is 'paralysing' the NHS (Daily Telegraph, 2023) due to the presence of too many 'inappropriate' elderly patients in NHS hospitals. Scott (2000) has argued that the 'bed blocking' label has created ageist attitudes towards older people in hospitals. They are seen as 'unwanted' and 'out of place' as the slower recovery of older people after surgery and acute illness renders them 'problem' patients (Mandelstam, 2011). Manzano-Santaella (2010) has suggested that a concern with delayed discharge originated with doctors but has increasingly been pursued on economic grounds to improve NHS 'efficiency'. She suggests that this depends on a narrow model of efficiency, since decelerating the care of older people can lead to better long-term outcomes, while accelerating hospital discharge can push a greater proportion of older patients into permanent residential care. She also suggests that measurement of delayed discharge is subjective, since the decision of clinicians to declare a patient 'medically fit' for discharge is affected by organisational context, particularly the pressure on clinicians to free up beds. Thus, she argues that the concept of bed-blocking is a 'complex fabrication' based on a socially constructed boundary between 'medical' needs and 'social' needs. As a consequence, the role of nurses has changed to give a high priority to the administrative work of socially constructing this boundary through the management of patient discharge (see Chapter 9).

In an ethnographic study of an acute medical ward, Latimer (2000) described nurses as **'conductors'** of care whose main job is to maintain organisational 'flow'. Latimer describes how flow is achieved by a continuous process of categorising and re-categorising patients. It is this process that socially constructs the boundary between 'medical' and 'social' needs. Older patients who do not follow an expected trajectory are progressively redefined as 'social' problems. They start to be seen as out of place and as polluting the purity of the medical domain (Douglas, 2003). There is hence a pressure to demedicalise their problems (Latimer, 1997). Below is a summary of a case example from her study:

Case Example: The Social Construction of a 'Social Admission'

Mrs Adamson (aged 84) is admitted with a diagnosis of a myocardial infarction, left ventricular failure and atrial fibrillation. Her stay involves several stages moving from 'high dependency' to 'observation' and then 'mobilisation'. From the outset the consultant keeps in play both a medical and a social interpretation of her problems. Alongside her medical diagnosis she is labelled as excessively anxious rendering her medical identity ambiguous. Over time she fails to make the required progress on the prescribed patient 'pathway'; she 'should' be getting better but is not. The 'social' label is brought to the fore; she is no longer described as having cardiac symptoms but 'odd turns' which are treated as medically ambiguous. She is being reconstituted as a 'social' case that is no longer the hospital's responsibility. She is now 'disposable' and is discharged to a home but readmitted two days later. On readmission she is not treated as an acute cardiac case but is described as a 'social' admission and mobilised with a view to discharge. She dies of a cardiac arrest on the bathroom floor two days later.

(LATIMER, 1997)

Several authors have suggested that the construction of older people as unwanted patients has negatively affected their experience of care. Oliver (2008) has suggested that older people deserve better than to be labelled as 'social admissions' and that frail, older people deserve better care, but instead frailty is treated as a disposal category. Oliver blames what he sees as poor treatment of older patients on prestige bias; doctors see caring for older people as low status and boring and this is linked to ageism in healthcare. Tomkow et al. (2023) have argued that the use of frailty scores to determine access to intensive care during the COVID-19 pandemic has further legitimated ageist rationing decisions which exclude older people from acute care.

We looked at patient labelling in Chapter 6. Maben (2012) found that a poor work environment combined with nurses' ageist attitudes led to labelling which negatively affected the experience of older people. Desirable patients were compliant and grateful and were labelled 'poppets', while patients who made demands were 'nuisances'. Maben says nurses' attitudes were not lost on patients who described themselves as being treated like 'parcels' bundled from one place to another as if they were objects, not people. Similarly, Tadd et al. (2011) found that older people were subjected to frequent ward moves in an attempt to accelerate their exit. They describe stark differences in the provision of dignified care for older people and highlight many examples of undignified care. Underpinning poor care was an **'othering'** of older people. There was a shared belief among staff that the older person (however acutely ill) was in the 'wrong' place and that there must be a better place for 'them' to be. Tadd and others conclude that their findings indicated widespread, entrenched ageism within NHS institutional culture.

Finally, an ethnographic study by Waring and Bishop (2019) described how older people experienced hospital discharge as an undignified, inhumane and unsafe process. Waring and Bishop characterised hospital discharge as the social production of **'bare life'**. The concept of 'bare life' comes from the Italian philosopher Giorgio Agamben. He defines 'bare life' as a **'state of exception'** in which people are rendered 'ineligible' and deprived of any citizenship rights or agency over their own life. People condemned to 'bare life' are those denied social rights; for example, people in refugee camps (Agamben, 2017). Patients in Waring et als' study were often discharged home without care being arranged, aids provided or adequate medication dispensed. Some were provided with wound dressings or injection kits without any help or instruction in how to use them. Waring and Bishop suggested that the 'health state of exception', which produced a condition of 'bare life' among older patients leaving the hospital, resulted from a complex health maze in which patients were passed back and forth between different agencies. These agencies were slow and bureaucratic and, after a period of time, each institution in turn decided that the older patient was an 'exception' to their rules and ineligible for help. The consequence was that no one was willing to take responsibility for their care, and they were abandoned to fend for themselves. The Health and Care Act 2022 (see Chapter 8) now allows hospitals to 'discharge to assess' patients so patients no longer need to have their care needs assessed before leaving the hospital. This is likely to worsen the situation described by Waring and Bishop.

Drawing on Bourdieu's theories of class (see Chapter 2), Kvael and Gautun (2023) have suggested that there are social inequalities in people's ability to negotiate this health maze. Patients and their families with greater economic, social and cultural capital know how to play the game to access better care and so these more privileged patients are more able to avoid 'bare life'.

REFLECTION POINT

Consider the definition of ageism above. Then look at the case example above. Do you think this was an example of ageism? How would you justify your opinion? Can you think of examples of ageism in healthcare or social care that you have seen or heard of in practice? Why do you think such ageism occurs? List your own ideas about how we could combat ageism in healthcare?

FAILURES IN HOSPITAL CARE

The most prominent hospital failure in recent years has been the scandal involving the Mid-Staffordshire Foundation NHS Trust. This case involved serious organisational failings over a lengthy period (2005–2008). Nurses at Mid-Staffordshire had failed to deliver the fundamentals of care such as basic hygiene and nutrition, and patients had suffered neglect and abuse; it was inferred that many may have died as a result. Neglect had been serious and systemic and nurses had failed to deliver safe and compassionate care (Francis, 2013). Amongst key recommendations by Robert Francis were the need for openness and candour throughout the healthcare system; named clinicians in charge of a patient's care; regulation of healthcare assistants and an organisational culture that supported compassionate care.

Institutional neglect in NHS hospitals had been seen before. The 1960s and 1970s saw frequent national enquiries into negligent care in NHS institutions, relating largely to the long-term care of elderly patients and patients with mental health problems (Martin, 1984). There are some marked similarities between these inquiries and the Mid-Staffordshire enquiry, particularly in respect to the neglect of the fundamentals of nursing care. What was different in the Mid-Staffordshire case was the occurrence of these deficiencies in an acute general hospital. One common denominator between these recent reports and earlier inquiries was that the victims were people who society often treats as having 'low social value', that is, they were mainly older and disabled people (Wardhaugh & Wilding, 1993). Although members of care staff were working in acute services, the populations subject to neglectful care were those same groups of older and disabled people who had featured in earlier inquiries.

Given the large number of inquiries that have taken place into poor institutional care it could be asked why lessons have not been learned and why the same problems occur repeatedly. Wardhaugh and Wilding (1993) produced an analysis of what they called the **'corruption of care'**. They concluded that the corruption of care depends on unthinking obedience to institutional demands coupled with the neutralisation of what the philosopher, Hannah Arendt, called 'animal pity' (Bergen, 2000). When care is corrupted, our capacities to both feel and think have been eroded. This depends on processes of depersonalisation through which people come to be **'othered'** and seen as less than fully human. Wardhaugh and Wilding suggested that certain client groups are particularly vulnerable to this dehumanising treatment. These are people who are seen as less than fully sentient as a result of their age and/or disabilities. It is these groups who are often viewed as 'out of place' in acute care. Negative labelling paves the way to poor care and unacceptable treatment. Wardhaugh and Wilding believed that the low social value attributed to some groups by both the institution and the wider culture devalued them in the eyes of care staff.

Wardhaugh and Wilding also suggested that the corruption of care is related to the dynamics of power and powerlessness in organisations. While victims of institutional abuse are frequently powerless and without a voice, they also noted that institutional abuse is more likely to occur in institutions where staff themselves feel powerless. Care is more likely to fail in closed, inward-looking institutions where ward staff are professionally isolated and have no voice. They suggest that failures in care are always underpinned by managerial failure, particularly a managerial culture that gives primacy to institutional efficiency.

Wardhaugh and Wilding believed that another key feature of the corruption of care was the disconnect between official rhetoric as expressed in an institution's policies and the 'sharp reality' of practice. Official policy might be full of idealistic objectives but the distribution of resources often demonstrated how far the institution fell short of its ideals. Resource allocation demonstrated the lack of value placed on certain patient groups; for example, when nurses in care of the elderly wards faced poor staffing levels and a lack of basic resources such as laundry. Thus, Wardhaugh and Wilding believed that the corruption of care could not be fixed by simply changing organisational culture. The distribution of power and resources within institutions also needed to change.

Walker (2012) has argued that ageism is built into health and social care policies at the highest levels of government. This can undermine care standards. This was starkly exposed during the COVID-19 pandemic (Carney et al., 2024). Martin (1984) suggested that policymakers use fine words, but the resources provided to care for certain populations, such as the elderly and learning disabled, contradict these fine words. Where resources are poor, staff may struggle to maintain high standards of care. While some staff experience moral distress in these circumstances (Maben, 2012), over time, depersonalised care can become normalised.

REFLECTION POINT

After reading this section, summarise the reasons for poor care, patient neglect and abuse. What do you think should be done to prevent these failures in care? How do you think you could help to prevent failures in care as an individual working in health and social care?

Care in the 'Community'

WHAT DO WE MEAN BY 'COMMUNITY CARE?'

According to Williams (2014), the word **community** dates back to the fourteenth century. It conjures a group of people who are directly and immediately related to one another and have something in common. This is usually related to locality. Williams says community is a 'warmly persuasive word' and thus is often associated with an imagined ideal community characterised by mutual understanding, mutual support and common feeling.

Much of the writing on communities since the twentieth century has mourned the passing of different types of community, such as the rural village (Blythe, 2005) or industrial communities disrupted by the decline of industries such as coal mining (Turner, 2000). Sociological theories of community have often focused on this decline. In the nineteenth century, people first began to notice the decline of traditional communities; in 1845, Prime Minister, Benjamin Disraeli, said that 'modern society acknowledges no neighbour' (Disraeli, 2017, p. 64). During this period, the German sociologist, Ferdinand Tonnies, described community (he called it **'gemeinschaft'**) as associated with 'kinship, neighbourhood and friendship'. He contrasted this with the new way of living (particularly in cities) that he called 'association' (or **'gesellschaft'**). He described 'association' as a feature of individualistic societies. Here, social ties were weakened and relationships were often contractual and dominated by rational calculation (Nisbet, 1993).

Thus, we can see modern societies as places where community ties in the old sense of kinship, neighbourhood and friendship may still exist but have been significantly weakened. For example, many people no longer live near their families or the place where they grew up. Thirteen percent of the UK population now live alone and over half of these people are over 65 years of age (ONS, 2023a). Local communities are often precarious, threatened and subordinate to political and economic forces; for example, the forces of globalisation can destroy industries at a stroke, hollowing out the communities that have depended on them for generations (Turner, 2000). It is ironic, therefore, that the word **'community'** plays such a prominent part in how policymakers talk about care outside of the hospital. The term 'community care' invites us to imagine community as a place where 'kinship, neighbourhood and friendship' still offer a reassuring web of support. The reality is often very different.

THE DEVELOPMENT OF CARE IN THE COMMUNITY

Most care outside of the hospital is, and always has been, delivered by family members but it has been augmented by nursing care services since the dawn of nursing as a profession. According to Heggie (2011), the professions of district nursing and health visiting developed in the late Victorian period to deliver nursing and public health to the sick poor. Initially, these were charitable services but they were gradually taken over by local authorities. After the creation of the NHS, community nursing services, although part of the NHS, remained under the control of local authority public health departments until the 1970s. Personal care in the home was delivered by the district nursing service with nursing assistants (supervised by district nurses) employed to deliver some of the fundamentals of care such as bathing. Like all NHS services, care was free. Social service departments delivered some means-tested 'social care' services such as 'meals on wheels' services and 'home helps' (home helps provided domestic help, such as cleaning and shopping). Social services departments also oversaw local authority-run residential homes and day centres (Thane, 2009). Thus, the boundary between health and social care was radically different to that which exists today and community nursing services played a much more central role in the care of the sick and frail in their own homes.

Case Example: District Nursing Before The Griffiths Community Care Reforms

Morrison (2017) carried out an oral history of community nursing services in the Outer Hebrides between the 1940s and 1970s. Community nurses played a pivotal role in the local community. In remote communities, 'triple duty' nurses acted as district nurse, midwife and health visitor. Here is an example of their work:
'When I started on my district there was a man very ill with chest cancer and I had to go to him daily and manage a chest drain which could be difficult. He was my first patient and after that the rest were just ordinary patients requiring general nursing care. If people were bedridden they had to be washed, toenails cut—no podiatrist then on the island. You really did what was necessary, changing beds, that sort of thing. With terminally ill patients, I often stayed with them all night especially if they were elderly and there was nobody else with them. I dressed the body when they died' (p. 82).

CHANGES IN THE ORGANISATION OF COMMUNITY CARE

At the end of the 1980s, Margaret Thatcher invited the businessman, Roy Griffiths, to follow up his review of NHS management (see Chapter 8) with a review of community care services.

The Griffiths review of community care dramatically changed the landscape of community care; creating a private market for residential and home care and redefining personal care in the home as 'social care' rather than 'nursing care'. This changed the role of community nursing services; redefining them as 'case managers' rather than providers of care (Pickard, 2009). According to Bramwell et al. (2023), this was an unwelcome expansion of their role away from care provision. From the 1980s onwards, community nurses also faced larger caseloads due to the drive to discharge patients from the hospital earlier and while sicker.

The main driver for the Griffiths review of community care was Thatcher's desire to cut care costs. Prior to his reforms, the benefits regulations allowed people in care homes to obtain supplementary pensions to pay for their board and lodgings. The bill for this had increased sharply to £280 million pounds (Hansard, 1986). Thatcher wanted to reduce these costs (Timmins, 2017). Griffiths put social services departments in charge of deciding people's eligibility for care; both in the home and in residential settings. This gave social workers a new role as care managers. This was a statutory responsibility which local authorities had to deliver by law, meaning 'social care' spending had to take priority over spending on non-statutory services such as libraries and community centres. The new system was cash limited to reduce costs. As a result, assessments of people's eligibility for help had to be tailored to the funds available rather than need. The numbers of people receiving funded support dropped significantly after the reforms.

Griffiths was also keen to encourage the development of the private sector in delivering what was now to be called 'social care'. The new private home care services employed unqualified care assistants rather than more expensive nurses. Over time, purchasing from these private companies largely replaced local authority-run services. Once personal care in the home was rebadged as 'social care' rather than 'nursing care', it could be means tested so that all but the poorest would be expected to pay for their care. Thus, older people and their families could face enormous care costs for care that would have once been provided free by the NHS.

Many found the new distinction between health and social care 'hopelessly blurred' (Griffiths, 1998). The new system created financial incentives to rebadge ever more complex care in the home as 'social care' and, over time, more care crossed the boundary from the health domain to the 'social care' domain. Social care spending began to swallow a larger and larger proportion of local authority budgets. Struggles developed between health and social care authorities, both seeking to avoid financial responsibility for older and disabled people needing ongoing care (Bridgen & Lewis, 1999). As a result, since the Griffiths reforms, social care for older people has consistently been viewed as being in crisis (Williams, 2021). This sense of crisis intensified in the era of austerity following the 2008 global financial crisis. Many local authorities were forced to ration social care to only those in the direst need (O'Hara, 2015).

Although attempts have been made to introduce 'partnerships' and 'integration' between health and social care, there have been systemic barriers to joined-up working, particularly in relation to finance (Bramwell et al., 2023). A key barrier is the distinction between free NHS care and means-tested social care. In Scotland, free social care for people over 65 years of age was introduced in 2002. Subsequent reforms have promoted more integration between health and social care in Scotland though funding issues remain problematic (Hendry et al., 2021). It seems that free social care (along with adequate funding) may be an essential step to end haggling over budgets and promote the integration of health and social care. Free social care has the potential to significantly improve the health of older and disabled people. However, other parts of the UK have yet to follow Scotland in offering free social care (Quilter-Pinner & Hochlaf, 2019). Pollock et al. (2020) have argued that we need a truly integrated national health and care service which reverses many of the changes made by Griffiths; bringing both services back under national control and making them publicly accountable.

INFORMAL CARE IN THE HOME

Most care in the home is carried out by unpaid workers. Where patients cannot carry out self-care, this involves care by family or friends. Often, care duties fall onto the shoulders of a single family member. As a result of the pressure to discharge patients early from the hospital, many more patients and their families now have to manage unfamiliar treatment tasks and technologies in the home (such as peritoneal dialysis), often with limited support. Informal carers in the UK engage in more intensive care, deliver longer hours of caring work and have more health problems than carers in countries that have more generous provisions for long-term care (Bom & Stockel, 2021). In the previous chapter, we considered the McDonaldisation of medicine, a key feature of which was 'putting the customer to work', and we can see McDonaldisation at work in the transfer of care and treatment tasks to patients and their families.

The Department of Health and Social Care (2018) defines informal care as someone who provides unpaid help to a friend or family member needing support due to illness, older age, disability or a mental health condition. According to Broese Van Groenou and De Boer (2016), governments are placing increasing reliance on informal carers as they cut back on professional care. Thus, the burdens on informal carers are increasing. They suggest that informal carers are motivated by values and affection but that they may face barriers to delivering care, such as geographical distance, employment demands, and financial and health difficulties. They also suggest that the decline in community support has impacted negatively on the ability of individuals to provide informal care.

The 2021 UK Census suggested that the total number of informal carers across all nations of the UK was 5.7 million people (ONS, 2023b). There are also approximately 800,000 young carers (aged 16 and under) in the UK. Roughly 60% of carers are females, and female carers are likely to be delivering longer hours of care than male carers. The 2021 census also showed that 30% of carers in England provided over 50 hours of care per week (Petrillo & Bennett, 2023). Just under half of carers are in employment, with three-quarters of working carers reporting that they struggled to juggle work and caring.

Caring negatively affects carers' incomes and also creates extra costs, such as heating. Two-thirds of carers in a recent survey said that that they were extremely worried about their finances, with ethnic minority carers reporting more financial difficulties (Carers UK, 2022). Perhaps unsurprisingly, carers have more physical and mental health problems than non-carers and are more likely to have unmet health needs. Musculoskeletal problems linked to the physical burden of caring are commonplace; one-third of carers have reported that their mental health is bad or very bad and half of all carers reported feeling lonely. Caring responsibilities can also lead to delays in carers getting their own health needs met; for example, carers may not be able to get respite care to attend outpatient appointments. Thus, Public Health England identified unpaid caregiving as an independent social determinant of ill health (Public Health England, 2021).

Support for carers fails to meet many carers' needs with more than a third of carers saying they had never received any support such as respite services. Many carers were also deterred from using support services due to high costs and dissatisfaction with standards of care (Carers UK, 2022). Carers have the right to ask for a carer's assessment to identify their need for support, but only 25% of carers in a recent survey had received one (Carers UK, 2022).

FORMAL CARE IN THE HOME

As we noted earlier, most personal care in the home is now defined as 'social care'. To receive any public funding towards 'social care' people must undergo a means test. Only someone with assets of less than £14,250 will receive free care while someone with assets of up to £23,500 will receive partial help on a sliding scale. Anyone with more than this will be expected to entirely fund their own care. The government has estimated that one in seven people over 65 years of age face a lifetime bill for care costs of over £100,000.

After the means test, a needs assessment determines whether people are considered to have sufficient needs to be entitled to care (King's Fund, 2023). Many older people face very long waits for assessments (Ward et al., 2022). Many care needs are unmet, and over a third of people applying to local authorities receive no help. Those that do receive help may receive a 'care package' which fails to meet all their needs as care is rationed due to funding pressures. Service users can also apply for 'personal budgets' to manage their own care but the numbers receiving these are very small and falling (Kings Fund, 2023). There is some NHS 'continuing care' funding for people with severe and complex long-term health needs, but the process for obtaining this is fraught with difficulty. The Parliamentary and Health Service Ombudsman (2020) has ruled that this system consistently fails the most vulnerable.

As we noted earlier, most paid care in the home is now provided by private companies commissioned by local authorities. Patient experience of this care is variable. A study by the Equality and Human Rights Commission (EHRC) looked at what older people valued about their care and also at where care failed. Older people valued care that preserved their independence, security, privacy and dignity. They valued care providers who provided continuity of care so they could build up a relationship with their care worker (EHRC, 2011). The EHRC identified many failings in social care at home. They concluded that these amounted to a breach of patients' human rights. These included: failing to provide adequate nutrition or help with eating; neglecting personal care; leaving tasks undone; patronising and ignoring the older person; failing to offer autonomy or choice; being inflexible in the timing of care (patients could be put to bed as early as 2:45pm); failing to respect clients' privacy and failing to respect the diverse needs of minority groups. One particularly common problem that they identified was that care companies operated with a defensive culture that led to staff hiding behind 'health and safety' to refuse to complete care tasks. The authors consulted the Health and Safety Executive who confirmed that this was unjustified. This could result in avoidable harms to patients, such as pressure sores. The Commission also identified instances of physical and financial abuse.

Examples: Good Versus Poor Home Care

Good care

"We have a good laugh which is what I need, they do the job, but we joke and laugh at the same time. It is important because when you are like us, you don't go out, you don't … see anybody. They are friends."

"The Council home care service is ultra-reliable, even in bad weather, and they are always cheerful … I have tremendous respect for the work they do."

Poor care

"In one incident an able-bodied, healthy 32-year-old female member of staff stood and watched as a 76-year-old woman with advanced cancer struggled from the lounge to the kitchen to microwave this dish herself, because the worker could not do this 'because of health and safety'.

"There were two care workers there, and they were talking to each other over the client, who was blind, completely ignoring him while they were assisting him…talking to each other while they're doing things to him, as if he's a lump of meat."

"Most of the girls [from the agency] were nasty; they were rough. Rather than say 'sit in the chair', they'd push me back into the chair, that sort of thing and I didn't like that … … I couldn't do anything about it. I can't even walk and I think they know this you see; they know you're vulnerable".

(EHRC, 2011)

Svanstrom et al. (2013) described community care as causing suffering when the care worker was task focused and not open to human contact with the care recipient. Objectifying the older person in this way eroded their sense of identity. This is similar to the 'corruption of care' described earlier. Ward et al. (2022) found that accessing social care meant losing 'temporal autonomy'. Decisions about the timing of visits and their duration were out of the hands of service users who had to accept that meal times, bed times etc. were no longer under their control. Tasks were timed and based on the company's 'clock' time; for example, 30- or 45-minute slots. Thus, time constraints on carers' visits could restrict other choices, such as over food and drink. Ward found that many people had to subsist solely on sandwiches or microwave meals that were quick to prepare within the carer's time slot. We can see in these examples that even people in receipt of care may be reduced to 'bare life' as described by Agamben (2017). Even though people receiving such care are living in their own homes, formal home care services can be organised in ways that greatly restrict a client's life and recreate the conditions of the total institution.

CARE HOMES

According to Kennedy (2014), we should all ask ourselves whether we would dread the prospect of ending our lives in a care home. If we find the prospect of life in a care home dreadful, he asks, what are we doing to change the situation? There were 372,000 people living in care homes in England alone in 2023, with numbers estimated at around half a million for all four countries in the UK. Thirty-seven percent of care home residents in England were paying for all or some of their care costs (Fox, 2023). One study found that most care home residents stayed for between one and three years (Forder & Fernandez, 2011). Two-thirds of care home residents are females, as are 95% of staff. Kennedy (2014) suggests that ageism and sexism pervade our attitudes to care homes. Care home workers are among the worst paid workers in the labour market.

Bowers et al. (2009) found that entry to a care home was usually abrupt and hurried, for example, following a hospital admission. Older residents felt that they had not been consulted about either the decision to go into a care home or given a choice of home, even when paying for their care. Being moved into a care home involves a significant loss of autonomy and human rights, with residents entirely at the mercy of the decisions of care home owners and managers. Residents had been forced to give up their homes, but once in a care home, had no security of tenure. Managers could terminate their residence at any time.

When asked by researchers, older people had clear ideas about what a good life in a care home would include; older people valued meaningful relationships, a personalised environment, individualised care, fulfilling activities and control over their daily lives (Bowers et al., 2009). Although some care homes are engaged in the local community, offer good care and provide meaningful activities for residents, many do not. Kennedy (2014) says that care homes could be the centre of their local community but are too often isolated from it, leaving their residents also isolated. Many care homes focus almost solely on physical care and operate within a defensive and risk-averse culture that limits the lives of their residents. This was starkly evident during the COVID-19 pandemic when residents were completely cut off from the outside world, including family; yet thousands of residents died from COVID-19 brought in by staff or by patients transferred in from hospitals (Daly, 2020).

The care provided within care homes can often resemble that of the total institutions with residents processed in batches according to rigid routines. For example, an ethnographic study of care homes found that staff worked with a production line model of care with the 'product' being the 'lounge ready' resident who could be wheeled out for display in the day room. The conditions and pace of work led to patients being treated as objects and facilitated 'bedroom abuse' with residents roughly handled and treated insensitively as they were processed (Lee-Treweek, 2008).

Care homes can be owned by public authorities, non-profit organisations or for-profit commercial companies. Ninety-five percent of care homes in the UK are now run by the private sector with increasing numbers run by large for-profit chains owned by private equity companies. For investors, the care home sector is highly profitable but these profits may be earned at the expense of standards of care. There is some evidence that for-profit homes are associated with worse care (Ronald et al., 2016). This is particularly true of the larger for-profit chains (Patwardhan et al., 2022). Many authors have called for radical reform of the long-term care sector both in respect to residential care and care in the home (Pollock et al., 2020). Despite a number of government reviews of care in the community, there is as yet little sign of the problems in the social care sector being adequately addressed. We can conclude therefore that there are serious deficiencies in community care services.

REFLECTION POINT

A number of studies have indicated that social care in the home can be poor and that there are gaps in services. Similar problems can exist in care homes. What do you think should be done to improve these services?

Summary of Key Points

- The hospital has changed as a result of policies designed to reduce inpatient care and increase ambulatory care. This has put a strain on both inpatient services and community services.
- There is institutional ageism in healthcare systems which can negatively affect the experiences of older patients as well as patient outcomes.
- The boundary between health and social care has changed with most care at home now delivered by private social care services. The social care system is complex; care is underfunded, and many sick and disabled people do not have their care needs met.
- There is increased use of private care homes for older patients. Care is often institutionalised and, in some cases, care standards are inadequate.

Further Reading

Lee-Treweek, G. (2008). Bedroom abuse: The hidden work in a nursing home. In Johnson, J., & De Souza, C. (Eds.), *Understanding health and social care: An introductory reader* (pp. 107–111). Sage Publications.

Maben, J., Adams, M., Peccei, R., Murrells, T., & Robert, G. (2012). 'Poppets and parcels': The links between staff experience of work and acutely ill older peoples' experience of hospital care. *International Journal of Older People Nursing, 7*(2), 83–94.

Morrison, C. (2017). *Hebridean Heroines: Twentieth century queen's nurses:1940s to 1970s.* Islands Book Trust.

Wardhaugh, J., & Wilding, P. (1993). Towards an explanation of the corruption of care. *Critical Social Policy, 13*(37), 4–31.

References

Agamben, G. (2017). *The omnibus homo sacer.* Stanford University Press.

Alotaibi, H. (2021). A review on the development of healthcare infrastructure through the history of Islamic civilization. *Journal of Healthcare Leadership, 13*, 139–145.

Armstrong, D. (1998). Decline of the hospital: Reconstructing institutional dangers. *Sociology of Health & Illness, 20*(4), 445–457.

Bergen, B. J. (2000). *The banality of evil: Hannah Arendt and 'the final solution.* Rowman & Littlefield Publishers.

Blythe, R. (2005). *Akenfield: Portrait of an English Village.* Penguin Books.

Bom, J., & Stöckel, J. (2021). Is the grass greener on the other side? The health impact of providing informal care in the UK and the Netherlands. *Social Science & Medicine, 269*, 113562.

Bowers, H. (2009). *Older people's vision for long term care*. Joseph Rowntree Foundation.

Bramwell, D., Checkland, K., Shields, J., & Allen, P. (2023). *Community nursing services in England: An historical policy analysis*. Springer Nature.

Bridgen, P., & Lewis, J. (1999). *Elderly people and the boundary between health and social care 1946–91: Whose responsibility?* Nuffield Trust.

Broese van Groenou, M. I., & De Boer, A. (2016). Providing informal care in a changing society. *European Journal of Ageing, 13*, 271–279.

Burtinshaw, K., & Burt, J. (2017). *Lunatics, imbeciles and idiots: A history of insanity in nineteenth-century Britain and Ireland*. Casemate Publishers.

Carers UK. (2022). *The state of caring*. Retrieved January 24, 2024, from. https://www.carersuk.org/media/p4kblx5n/cukstateofcaring2022report.pdf.

Carney, G. M., Maguire, S., & Byrne, B. (2024). 'Oldies come bottom of Grim Reaper hierarchy': A framing analysis of UK newspaper coverage of old age and risk of dying during the first wave of the COVID-19 pandemic. *Journal of Social Policy, 53*(3), 854–875.

Carney, T. (2008). The mental health service crisis of neoliberalism—An Antipodean perspective. *International Journal of Law and Psychiatry, 31*(2), 101–115.

Castagna, F., Xue, X., Saeed, O., Kataria, R., Puius, Y. A., Patel, S. R., & Jorde, U. P. (2022). Hospital bed occupancy rate is an independent risk factor for COVID-19 inpatient mortality: A pandemic epicentre cohort study. *BMJ Open, 12*(2), e058171.

Daily Telegraph (2023). The NHS must solve its bed-blocking crisis. Retrieved October 28, 2023, from https://www.telegraph.co.uk/opinion/2023/07/23/nhs-must-solve-its-bed-blocking-crisis/.

Daly, M. (2020). COVID-19 and care homes in England: What happened and why? *Social Policy & Administration, 54*(7), 985–998.

Department of Health and Social Care. (2018). *How can we improve support for carers?* Retrieved November 1, 2023, from. https://assets.publishing.service.gov.uk/government/uploads/system/uploads/attachment_data/file/713695/response-to-carers-call-for-evidence.pdf.

Dingwall, R., Rafferty, A. M, & Webster, C. (2002). *An introduction to the social history of nursing*. Routledge.

Disraeli, B. (2017). *Sybil or the two nations*. Oxford University Press.

Douglas, M. (2003). *Purity and danger: An analysis of concepts of pollution and taboo*. Routledge.

Englander, D. (2013). *Poverty and poor law reform in nineteenth-century Britain, 1834–1914: From Chadwick to Booth*. Routledge.

Equality and Human Rights Commission. (2011). *Close to home: An inquiry into older people and human rights in home care*. Retrieved January 24, 2024, from https://www.equalityhumanrights.com/sites/default/files/close_to_home.pdf.

Forder, J., & Fernandez, J.-L. (2011). *Length of stay in care homes* (pp. 2769). PSSRU Discussion Paper.

Foucault, M. (2002). *The birth of the clinic*. Routledge.

Foucault, M. (2019). *Discipline & punish: The birth of the prison*. Penguin Books.

Fox, A. (2023). *Number of care home residents in England rises in past year to more than 372,000*. The Independent.

Francis, R. (2013). *Report of the Mid Staffordshire NHS foundation trust public inquiry*. The Stationery Office.

Goffman, E. (2017). *Asylums: Essays on the social situation of mental patients and other inmates*. Routledge.

Gorsky, M. (2013). 'To regulate and confirm inequality'? A regional history of geriatric hospitals under the English National Health Service, c. 1948–c. 1975. *Ageing and Society, 33*(4), 598–625.

Griffiths, J. (1998). Meeting personal hygiene needs in the community: A district nursing perspective on the health and social care divide. *Health & Social Care in the Community, 6*(4), 234–240.

Hansard (1986). HC Deb 09 July 1986 vol 101 cc318–57. https://api.parliament.uk/historic-hansard/commons/1986/jul/09/residential-care-for-the-elderly

Heggie, V. (2011). Health visiting and district nursing in victorian manchester; divergent and convergent vocations. *Women's History Review, 20*(3), 403–422.

Hendry, A., Thompson, M., Knight, P., McCallum, E., Taylor, A., Rainey, H., & Strong, A. (2021). Health and social care reform in Scotland–what next? *International Journal of Integrated Care, 21*(4), 7.

Higginbottom, P. (2016). *The workhouse: The story of an institution*. Retrieved January 24, 2024, from. https://www.workhouses.org.uk/.

Jönson, H., & Taghizadeh Larsson, A. (2021). Ableism and ageism. In Gu, D., & Dupre, M. E. (Eds.), *Encyclopedia of gerontology and population aging* (pp. 4–9). Springer International.

Kennedy, J. (2014). *John Kennedy's care home inquiry*. Retrieved January 24, 2024, from. https://www.jrf.org.uk/careinquiry.

Kings Fund. (2023). *Social care in a Nutshell*. Retrieved January 24, 2024, from. https://www.kingsfund.org.uk/projects/nhs-in-a-nutshell/social-care-nutshell.

Kvæl, L. A. H., & Gautun, H. (2023). Social inequality in navigating the healthcare maze: Care trajectories from hospital to home via intermediate care for older people in Norway. *Social Science & Medicine, 333*, 116142.

Latimer, J. (2000). *The conduct of care: Understanding nursing practice*. Wiley-Blackwell.

Latimer J. (1997). Giving patients a future: The constituting of classes in an acute medical unit. Sociology of Health & Illness, *19*(2), 160–185.

Lee-Treweek, G. (2008). Bedroom abuse: The hidden work in a nursing home. In Johnson, J., & De Souza, C. (Eds.), *Understanding health and social care: An introductory reader* (pp. 107–111). Sage Publications.

Levy, S., & Apriceno, M. (2019). Ageing: The role of ageism. *OBM Geriatrics, 3*(4), 83.

Maben, J., Adams, M., Peccei, R., Murrells, T., & Robert, G. (2012). Poppets and parcels': The links between staff experience of work and acutely ill older peoples' experience of hospital care. *International Journal of Older People Nursing, 7*(2), 83–94.

Mandelstam, M. (2011). *How we treat the sick: Neglect and abuse in our health services*. Jessica Kingsley Publishers.

Manzano-Santaella, A. (2010). From bed-blocking to delayed discharges: Precursors and interpretations of a contested concept. *Health Services Management Research, 23*(3), 121–127.

Martin, J. P. (1985). *Hospitals in trouble*. Wiley-Blackwell.

McDonald, L. (Ed.). (2012). *Florence nightingale and hospital reform: Collected works of Florence Nightingale*, 16. Wilfrid Laurier University Press.

McLaughlin, K. (2020). Recognising elderspeak and how to avoid its use with older people. *Mental Health Practice, 26*(4), 6.

Morrison, C. (2017). *Hebridean heroines: Twentieth century queen's nurses:1940s to 1970s*. Islands Book Trust.

Nisbet, R. A. (1993). *The sociological tradition*. Transaction Publishers.

O'Hara, M. (2015). *Austerity bites: A journey to the sharp end of cuts in the UK*. Policy Press.

Office of National Statistics (ONS). (2023). *Families and households in the UK: 2022*. Retrieved January 24, 2024, from. https://www.ons.gov.uk/peoplepopulationandcommunity/birthsdeathsandmarriages/families/bulletins/familiesandhouseholds/2022#:~:text=The%20number%20of%20people%20living,households%20were%20women%20living%20alone.

Oliver, D. (2008). 'Acopia' and 'social admission' are not diagnoses: Why older people deserve better. *Journal of the Royal Society of Medicine, 101*(4), 168–174.

ONS. (2023). *Unpaid care, England and Wales: Census 2021*. Retrieved January 24, 2024, from. https://www.ons.gov.uk/peoplepopulationandcommunity/healthandsocialcare/healthandwellbeing/bulletins/unpaidcareenglandandwales/census2021#:~:text=In%20England%20and%20Wales%20an,2011%20to%204.4%25%20in%202021.

Oxford English Dictionary. (2023). *'asylum ear, n.'*. Oxford University Press. Retrieved January 24, 2024, from. https://doi.org/10.1093/OED/8881805545.

Parliamentary and Health Service Ombudsman. (2020). *NHS continuing healthcare failing to provide care for most vulnerable, says Ombudsman*. Retrieved January 24, 2024, from. https://www.ombudsman.org.uk/news-and-blog/news/nhs-continuing-healthcare-failing-provide-care-most-vulnerable-says-ombudsman#:~:text=Complaints%20to%20the%20Ombudsman%20about,for%20a%20family%20member's%20care.

Patwardhan, S., Sutton, M., & Morciano, M. (2022). Effects of chain ownership and private equity financing on quality in the English care home sector: Retrospective observational study. *Age & Ageing, 51*(12), 222.

Pepper, C. (2015). Person-centered communication: Ageism—The core problem. In Storlie, T. (Ed.), *Person-centered communication with older adults: The professional provider's guide* (pp. 73). Academic Press.

Petersen, A. (2012). Foucault, health and healthcare. In Scambler, G. (Ed.), *Contemporary theorists for medical sociology* (pp. 7–20). Routledge.

Petrillo, M., & Bennett, M. R. (2023). *Valuing carers 2021: England and Wales*. Carers UK.

Pickard, S. (2009). Governing old age: The 'Case Managed' older person. *Sociology, 43*(1), 67–84.

Pollock, A. M., Clements, L., & Harding-Edgar, L. (2020). Covid-19: Why we need a national health and social care service. *BMJ, 369*, m1465.

Porter, R. (2004). *Blood and guts: A short history of medicine*. WW Norton & Company.

Public Health England. (2021). *Caring as a social determinant of health: Review of evidence.* Retrieved January 24, 2024, from. https://www.gov.uk/government/publications/caring-as-a-social-determinant-of-health-review-of-evidence.

Quilter-Pinner, H., & Hochlaf, D. (2019). *Social care: Free at the point of need—The case for free personal care in England.* Institute for Public Policy Research.

Ronald, L. A., McGregor, M. J., Harrington, C., Pollock, A., & Lexchin, J. (2016). Observational evidence of for-profit delivery and inferior nursing home care: When is there enough evidence for policy change? *PLoS Medicine, 13*(4), e1001995.

Scott, H. (2000). Elderly patients: People not 'bed-blockers. *British Journal of Nursing, 9*(9), 528.

Scull, A. T. (2014). *Decarceration: Community treatment and the deviant-a radical view.* John Wiley & Sons.

Selvan, F. (2012). In defence of small hospitals. 27th September. *Health Service Journal.*

Shermer, M. (2016). Why Malthus is still wrong. *Scientific American, 314*(5), 72.

Siverskog, J , & Henriksson, M. (2022). The health cost of reducing hospital bed capacity. *Social Science & Medicine, 313*(11), 5399.

Svanström, R., Sundler, A. J., Berglund, M., & Westin, L. (2013). Suffering caused by care—Elderly patients' experiences in community care. *International Journal of Qualitative Studies on Health and Well-being, 8*(1), 20603.

Tadd, W., Hillman, A., Calnan, S., Calnan, M., Bayer, T., & Read, S. (2011). *Dignity in practice: An exploration of the care of older adults in acute NHS trusts.* HMSO.

Thane, P. (2009). *Memorandum submitted to the House of Commons Health Committee Inquiry: Social care.* History and Policy. Retrieved January 24, 2024, from. https://www.historyandpolicy.org/docs/thane_social_care.pdf. Retrieved.

Timmins, N. (2017). *The five giants: A biography of the welfare state.* HarperCollins.

Tomkow, L., Pascall-Jones, P., & Carter, D. (2023). Frailty goes viral: A critical discourse analysis of COVID-19 national clinical guidelines in the United Kingdom. *Critical Public Health, 33*(1), 116–123.

Turner, R. (2000). *Coal was our life.* Sheffield Hallam University Press.

Walker, A. (2012). The new ageism. *The Political Quarterly, 83*(4), 812–819.

Ward, R., Rummery, K., Odzakovic, E., Manji, K., Kullberg, A., Keady, J., & Campbell, S. (2022). Taking time: The temporal politics of dementia, care and support in the neighbourhood. *Sociology of Health & Illness, 44*(9), 1427–1444.

Wardhaugh, J., & Wilding, P. (1993). Towards an explanation of the corruption of care. *Critical Social Policy, 13*(37), 4–31.

Waring, J., & Bishop, S. (2020). Health states of exception: Unsafe non-care and the (inadvertent) production of 'bare life' in complex care transitions. *Sociology of Health & Illness, 42*(1), 171–190.

Weir, K. (2023). Ageism is one of the last socially acceptable prejudices. Psychologists are working to change that. *Monitor on Psychology, 54*(2), 36.

Williams, F. (2021). *Social policy: A critical and intersectional analysis.* Polity Press.

Williams, R. (2014). *Keywords: A vocabulary of culture and society.* Oxford University Press.

World Health Organization. (2022). Abuse of older people. World Health Organization. Retrieved January 24, 2024, from. https://www.who.int/news-room/fact-sheets/detail/elder-abuse.

INDEX